Eagles, Angels and Butterflies

How We Got Our Wings

TONYA T. GRIFFIN

Bloomington, IN 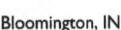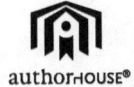 Milton Keynes, UK

authorHOUSE®

AuthorHouse™
1663 Liberty Drive, Suite 200
Bloomington, IN 47403
www.authorhouse.com
Phone: 1-800-839-8640

AuthorHouse™ UK Ltd.
500 Avebury Boulevard
Central Milton Keynes, MK9 2BE
www.authorhouse.co.uk
Phone: 08001974150

This book is a work of non-fiction. Unless otherwise noted, the author and the publisher make no explicit guarantees as to the accuracy of the information contained in this book and in some cases, names of people and places have been altered to protect their privacy.

First published by AuthorHouse 9/11/2006

ISBN: 1-4259-4844-8 (sc)

Printed in the United States of America
Bloomington, Indiana

This book is printed on acid-free paper.

Foreward

🦋

*G*od is the Author and Finisher of my faith and this book. He is also my Editor in Chief. Thank you God for giving me a life worth writing about.

Most people look at cancer as a death sentence, and in many cases they're right. Whenever, I tell people that I am a 15-year, two-time, 36 year-old breast cancer survivor that refused chemotherapy, they look at me initially as if I'd slapped them. Then they immediately begin to hear Gregorian-Chant Music in the background like I have just sprouted wings. It can be quite amusing to watch some-times.

This book is dedicated to all the cancer survivors out there. <u>We</u> <u>are</u> <u>butterflies</u>. I consider myself a butterfly, be-cause my Mom says that I am beautiful, strong and free. Eagles are those survivors who have been able to soar far beyond my mere accomplishments, and gone on to become great orators, lobbyists or advocates for the cancer cause. Angels were survivors first, they have since finished their work on this earth, and their spirits have gone back to the God that gave it.

Many people believe that if you have survived cancer, especially after a certain number of years have passed, life should be a gravy boat at this point. That couldn't be further from the truth. Some of my most trying days in my life had nothing to do with cancer. This is a diary of surviving <u>life</u>, after surviving cancer. You will notice that the events of some days are not recorded. These days <u>do</u> hold significance to me personally, but only a fool speaks <u>all</u> his mind.

My prayer is that something in this book will inspire you to ask God to heal your life.

Dedications

To my loving husband, you are my knight-in-shining-armor, my friend and my confidante. I love you more than you can know...you inspire me daily. To my beautiful little girls, Taylor Allison and Reyna Ezella, both of you are gifts from God and having you in my life pushes me to live and live, and live some more. I love you. To my wonderful parents...any good in me I attribute to God leading you to be the best parents you could be to me. I am forever grateful to you Ma and Daddy and I love you more than words can express. To my brothers and sisters - Moda, Jamison, D, Weezer and Jessi Bea...there were 6 of us growing up so things got hairy at times, but when I look back at our times together, I can do nothing but smile. You are each geniuses in your own rite and I am so proud you call me "sister." I love you to the ends of the earth. To my Uncle Mike...your life is a testimony of what God can do...you don't even have to say a word...your mere presence in my life inspires me to walk with God...Thank You. To my dear friends, Kim, Eric and kids...you always keep me laughing, and laughter is great medicine. To Charmean, we've been friends for more than 25 years, and you still make me laugh so hard I cry. I thank God for what he's doing in your life. To Yella, I'm so proud of all you have accomplished, and I'm glad we can share the trials and triumphs of motherhood, and laugh about it. And finally and most significantly...to the Master of My Universe, the Lover and Keeper of My Soul, my Lord and Savior Jesus Christ...what can I say Lord...it's all you, Father...it's all you.

*S*o far I'm having a decent day. Taylor's not whining too much and she's not insisting on being held all day. I wanted to talk about the word scary. S-C-A-R-Y. The significance of that word in my life is this. When you've had a lot of things go terribly wrong early in your life you tend to be more fearful than someone who has not experienced the same thing. For example, I had a less than pleasant experience in day-care and with sitters. Therefore I am literally petrified of leaving my baby with non-relatives (and there's some relatives I'd think twice about also). You get my drift? I'll try to use one of my least bone-chilling experiences. I remember when I was about 3 or 4 my cousin and I attended the same day-care. He was a typical 3 or 4 year-old running around, being a smart mouth at times…and he hadn't quite mastered the whole pee-pee-in-the-potty phenomenon. So from time to time he didn't smell as "April Fresh" as some of the other kids. I felt the day-care workers had it in for him. Well, anyway, he was acting up one afternoon and I guess the day-care workers had had enough. They took the flat part of a Webster's Dictionary and whomped him on the top the head. And yes, it was a hardback! I was stupefied and mortified all at the same time. Now this incident happened back in 1974. So what in the name of all that is holy, do you think is going

1

on in day-cares across the country here today?! I don't even want to think about it because as I said before, this was one of my <u>least</u> bone-chilling experiences.

Wednesday, October 2, 2002 8:07 AM

✦

I was thinking last night about something I wanted to talk about today, but now I can't remember…oh well. I'm supposed to have lunch with some former co-workers tomorrow, but I really have to play it by ear since Taylor has a bad cough. I'm unsure if I want to give her decongestants or not. I try to avoid giving her drugs at all cost, because the funny thing about our society is that someone has to die before they decide that a drug is unsafe. I like for them to work out all the kinks of a drug before I give it to my child. I guess I'm just cautious that way, call me crazy. I wanted to talk more about Taylor and day-care. I left my career to come home to be with my baby girl. I just don't want to have any regrets concerning her. I don't want to be one of those mothers who end up saying… "I wish I had been there for my child's first step." "I wish I had been there for the formative years, because I never got a chance to help shape his personality." Well maybe they won't say those exact words, but you know what I'm saying. And you know what? Ever since I took my sabbatical, I teeter back and forth on whether I made the right decision, and I'll tell you why. Money! Money! Money! Money! The economy is horrible right now and we're not bringing in half of what we use to. So we are cutting corners everywhere to make ends meet and not have to change our zip code. It has not been

3

easy but it's been 6 months since I left the workforce and we haven't lost anything nor have we starved. Thank God for that! That's one issue. The other issue is my adjustment to motherhood. Sometimes I look at my baby and wonder… "Lord, what were you thinking when you gave me a child to tend to for at least the next 18 years?" To think I'm directly responsible for the person she is to become almost blows my mind. But I take it one day at a time like the many mothers before me, while I pray constantly for guidance and strength. This is by far the hardest thing I have ever done in my life. Phew! It's almost overwhelming. I thought my bout with the "Big C" would be the most challenging thing I'd ever encounter, but God in his sovereignty said "Baby, you ain't seen nothing yet!" But anything worth having has a cost attached to it, and I can't imagine my life without her nor do want to. She's truly a blessing from God…literally. I remember a year or so before she was conceived I had the most vivid dream. I was walking near my favorite grocery store and it was the clearest, most beautiful day I'd ever seen. I was crossing the street and it was like time stood still. There were no cars, no people; the wind wasn't even blowing. All of a sudden I heard a sound from above, so I looked up into the baby blue sky. There was this "object" that penetrated the heavens with a sucking sound; it drove through the atmosphere with a sonic boom. Then, it hit the ground with a thud, but the asphalt immediately turned into rubber and the thing bounced up, and then landed back on the ground. I looked at this falling star, this thing, this extraterrestrial. It was a beautiful, bubbly, bouncing baby girl. She had round cheeks like a chipmunk, pink lips like rose petals, long beautiful eyelashes, and a wondrous God-given tan that would last a lifetime. SHE WAS MY BABY GIRL!! I picked her up, told her how beautiful she was and walked away with her in my arms. So now you understand when I tell you…my baby was <u>sent to me</u>, special delivery, from God himself.

Thursday, October 3, 2002 8:05 AM

❦

*T*oday is a halfway decent day so far...Taylor is not feeling well and neither am I. We're both fighting a bad cough, and I'm not sure if she gave it to me or I gave it to her or if we caught it at the same time. Well it's a moot point at this stage so let's talk about something more interesting. Let's talk about how chronic childhood illnesses affect you as an adult. When I was born, I had chronic asthma. It was so bad at birth, that I had to spend the first weeks of my life in an oxygen tent, according to my mother. I know what you're thinking, the girl in the plastic bubble...well that was me. My mother told me how upset she was that she couldn't touch me except through the gloves made on the side of the tent for people to reach through. Now I have no idea what was running through my brand new mind at this time but I can only imagine. Growing up I had to be careful not to send myself into an asthmatic episode. So when the humidity and pollen count were high during those steamy summer days in the Ohio-Valley, while my friends were outside playing kickball or getting sprayed with the waterhose, I had to be inside. I also couldn't get excited because I would immediately start coughing like a whooping crane or wheezing like a baby pig. "Stop fanning around," my mother would say so I would keep still. So there you have it. There was a constant sense of fear, surrounding my existence because of my poor health. But I guess one day my mother had had enough. She was tired of rushing me to the emergency room due to close calls. She was tired of watching me get poked and prodded by a series of physicians that may or may not have known what they were doing. She was tired of watching me take pills everyday and carry my inhaler like a magic pistol. I'm imagining she was like Popeye. "She had had all she could stand…" I will never forget what happened next as long as I live. I was 6 years old and had recently had one of many "near death experiences." My Mom took me to one of those old-fashioned Wednesday-Night Prayer Meetings. When the time came she took me up front to a beautiful gray-haired lady and told her my condition. The old woman got out some smelly oil, made a cross on my head with it, and proceeded to pray for me. My mother was praying too. Then they were done. The next day I was supposed to be taking a nap and my mother came in her bedroom, where I was bouncing up and down on her bed. She handed me her old torn up Bible. She opened it to Isaiah 53, where the scripture says "…he was wounded for our transgressions, he was bruised for our iniquities, the chastisement for our peace was upon him, and with is stripes we are healed." She had me read it over and over. Well I read this passage until I had it memorized. (You'll see later how that scripture came in handy later on in my life.) And from that day until this, I have never, ever, ever had another asthma attack. The pills and the inhaler…I don't know exactly when we threw them out, but we did. Some say I just grew out of it…I beg to differ.

Friday, October 4, 2002 8:22 AM

You know what? Today I am tired. I'm tired of poo poo diapers and whining. I'm tired of a lot of things. But the thing I am most tired of is <u>me</u>. I'm tired of living my life through the eyes and expectations of others...I'm tired of the fat I still have on my body that has nothing to do with giving birth. I'm tired of bills and bottles. I'm just tired. You know what amazes me? It's called the male species. You remember the phrase "Men are from Mars..." I beg to differ. I think Mars is a bad analogy, because Mars is in our solar system. I think men are from a planet in a totally different galaxy...maybe Ork or Vega. For example, a little over a week ago I put on a really nice, new dress. It showed all my curves, yet it was still a classy and stylish fit. I put the dress on, even had my toenails polished with a little toe-ring on. Now, it's been a while since E.T. saw me look this good (and I know I was looking good), since I had recently lost another 15 lbs., in addition to losing all the weight I had gained from the pregnancy. I looked wonderful, I smelled great, and had the confidence of a peacock and strutted accordingly. Do you know "Mork" didn't even notice? If he did he certainly didn't let me know. But that's ok, because me, and every person I ran into that day, knew I was looking exceptional.

Saturday, October 5, 2002 10:43 AM

✦

I feel like a prisoner in my own home!!! Taylor is going through her separation anxiety phase and it's driving me bonkers. I have to be near her at all times or she goes ballistic. She cries, she screams, she throws herself down so I have to pick her up or come to get her. But it's Saturday and that's always a good thing because it's a lazy day for ev-erybody. People aren't trying to kill you on the road to make it to their destination. Nobody's complaining about work because Saturday is the day you can forget you even have a job, unless you're one of those poor souls that have to work the weekends too. Now that I'm an adult I fully understand the meaning behind the song. "Everybody's working for the weekend…. Everybody's going off the deep-end!" I don't feel very talkative today so, I'm going to leave it at that. In the words of my late Granny, "be good, but if you can't be good be careful."

Sunday, October 13, 2002 6:09 P.M.

🦋

I'm a little late getting started today but here I am nonetheless. I wanted to talk about body image, weight-loss, and beauty or the lack thereof. Over my 32 years I have seen myself at various stages of my life obsessed with body image. In my early teen years I remember the "summer of starvation." I wasn't really trying to starve myself; I just wanted to make sure I didn't go back to being the chubby little 6th grader I used to be. So that summer I would eat no breakfast, a few green beans for lunch and a sensible dinner. I guess it was the equivalent to one of those skip-a-meal-plans, except the plans allow you drink a "filling, delicious shake." Yes, I'm being facetious but you get my drift. Well from age 14 to 28, I maintained my size 9, teetering every so often to a size 7. It was the perfect size for me, whenever I got smaller than that everyone said I looked sick, and I did. I was thinking yesterday that I didn't want to give you the wrong image...today I am a size 12. I hate being this size. I don't feel comfortable; therefore I've been training myself not to eat after a certain hour and to get exercise at least 4 times a week. The inches are dropping; I can tell in my clothes, but the scale JUST WON'T COOPERATE! I'm not going to get discouraged however, because even at a size 12...I look good. Let's go back to the "summer of starvation." My older sister had some teen magazine subscription, and I being the impressionable kid that I was, thought I was less than a person because I didn't look like the girls in the magazine. So I used deductive reasoning. I eat...therefore I'm fat...so I'll stop eating, as much. I never went through the bulimia or full fledge anorexia, but that's only because my family and friends, assured me that I had the perfect body weight for my height, and they were right. So I just exercised on a regular basis and went back to eating whatever I wanted.

🦋

*W*ell, I'm getting a late start again today, but I'm sure you could care less. Yesterday we were talking about weight and body image and all that hoopla. I was watching a show today that was talking about the very same subject. How we, as mothers, teach our daughters about body image, by what we do, and what we say about ourselves when we don't know their listening. What we say to them has far less impact than what we say about ourselves. As I was watching this I reflected on today's events. I was changing Taylor's diaper, and passed the mirror, noticing how this ponytail makes my head look huge and when I scrunch my head down a certain way, and I promise you I see another neck growing. In my disgust and discontent I said, "Gross…I look disgusting…I have to lose some more weight." Taylor looked at me as if to say…"who is this crazy lady talking to?" I smiled and assured her I wasn't talking about her, but myself. I really have got to do better. Thank God she doesn't understand me completely. But one day soon she will and I want to portray the right image. I don't want her to think that she has to be a supermodel to be loved, or accepted, or a good person. I don't want her to be as shallow as I have been. I look back on how my mother was when I was growing up. She had 6 kids and maintained a size 7 up until she had her tubes tied. She was about my age when she had it done. By the time her last child was 6 years old, my mother was a size 22. It was unbelievable to see. There were many other factors going on in her life that I won't get into. I'll let her write her own book for that. The gist of the matter was that she used food to bury her feelings and to comfort herself…a trait many women have. Feel sad? Let's bake some homemade chocolate chip cookies. Someone hurt your feelings? Let's go get some ice cream. I have a challenge for the men in the world. Make your size 18 woman feel good about herself by what you say and do. Mothers encourage your daughters to talk to you about anything they want…I mean anything. Fathers let your sons cry if they need to. It'll be a Dietary Revolution up in this piece!!! Do you know that there are now more obese people in our country than there have ever been in history? Do you think it's due to french-fries and white sugar? We've been eating sugar and fried potatoes for centuries… I tend to think there's more to it than that. People are very, very unhappy and dissatisfied with their lives. We as a society have emphasized money over all else. Now I might be starting a revolution when I say this, so I'll say it slow. Stop…working…for…money. Start working for you and the money will come. Working for you means doing the things you love…but let me clarify. If you love hurting yourself or anyone else, in any way…read my lips…I AIN'T TALKING TO YOU. I'm talking to the people who <u>don't</u> need to stop right now and seek professional help. I'm joking but I'm dead serious about that. I'm not down with people hurting other people. It's kinda a funny, my hubby called me a flowerchild earlier today. I don't know if he meant it as a compliment but it really made my day. I just want to be free. Free from letting the opinions of others sway me, free from my past failures, free from my own fears, free to grow an afro if I feel like it, free from the latest fads or trends, and free from Hollywood's personification of life or happiness. I just want to be free to be me, whoever I may be. I say that because I have not even scratched the surface of my potential or abilities. Please be patient with me…you know the rest. See ya. Oh by the way, my mother is a size 9 now. Go Ma!!!!

Wednesday, October 16, 2002 12:27 PM

❧

Sorry we didn't get to talk yesterday. I was having some technical difficulties. I was thinking this morning about the many people out there who are suffering with cancer. They're dealing with the torture of chemotherapy; and they're being burned at the stake by their radiation treatments. Then to add insult to injury they're being scalped a little every day in order for them to get "cured." I pray for them all the time. My heart bleeds for them because they are only following the advice of their doctors and for about 6 months to a year, their quality of life is zilch. Now, let me say this. I have the utmost respect for the medical profession. In fact if I could start my life all over again, I probably would have been a doctor. But when I was diagnosed with breast cancer at the tender age of 21, I told my doctor "No." She advised me to do about 6 months of chemotherapy and 6 weeks of radiation. I told her I'd do the radiation, but I said no to chemotherapy. She told me I could die and I said no again. She said, "You know you are acting against my medical advice." I said no again. Now I want you to understand something, prior to that day…I had never…in my life…done anything so reckless, so bold, so kamikaze. But something in the depths of my soul would not let me take the chemotherapy. I had done lots of research on the subject before I made my decision. I just couldn't do it…it just didn't make sense to me… at all. Let me get this straight. I'm going to kill all my white blood cells, the cells that God designed to fight against diseases, with this man-made stuff, all in the name of killing the cancer that may or may not come back anyway. It does not compute! It does not compute! Let me take my chances…if I have to die…and believe when I tell you, I don't want to die…but if I have to, I want to die on my on terms. I did take the radiation, but only for a couple of weeks. They kept drawing on me with this ugly, purple magic marker, which wasn't that bad. The bad part was the holes that were being burned into my skin and would not heal, because I was getting nuked <u>everyday</u>. I remember thinking, okay, now they've done it. I'm going to have to trust God, and my will to live completely now. "He was wounded for my transgressions, he was bruised for my iniquities, the chastisement for my peace was upon him, and with his stripes I am healed!" Remember I told you about this scripture when I was fighting asthma? It became my mantra. I quoted it everyday for about 5 years straight. I still quote it now. And each time I feel an ache or pain that Fear tells me is the cancer coming back, I quote that scripture. I've been doing this for almost 12 years now, and I'm still here…I'm still here.

Thursday, October 17, 2002 10:52 am

🦋

*T*was supposed to have lunch today with some former co-workers but one had to cancel. That worked out because we all overslept today. It's probably because my hubby is sick with a cold and kept everybody up all night coughing. I wanted to talk about something a little more upbeat today. I want to talk about living your dreams. Notice "dream" is plural, and there's a reason for it. Most people, if they really took the time to think about it, have several different dreams…some are interconnected and some are not. If you want to be mundane, you could call it a goal. Some…sorry, Taylor's eating my thesaurus…we'll continue this later, she must want breakfast.

Friday, October 18, 2002 8:01 pm

🦋

*O*kay, it's 8:00 pm and I finally get a moment to myself. I was thinking about what I wanted to talk to you about today. It's a subject I've tiptoed around for the past several days, but I think I'm ready to talk about it. It's friendship. I don't use the term freely because I don't call every Tom, Dick, and Harry my friend. I used to do that when I was younger and didn't know any better…but back then, I didn't know how to be a true friend either. A true friend will tell you the truth no matter how much it may hurt, while they do everything in their power not to hurt you. It's quite a feat. I've learned that a true friend loves you when you're poor, and they love you when you're rich. Now you may think…it's easy to love a rich friend, but that's not always the case. What if you and I grew up in the same neighborhood, went to the same school, got the same grades, and dated in some of the same circles. Now what if you, being my good friend, know all my flaws, idiosyncrasies and indiscretions. Now all of a sudden, I become rich. You hear other people sing my praises, simply because I'm rich. I'm not any more worthy of the wealth than you are, in fact. I shop at Barney's, your clothes make you look like Barney. My kid goes to private school; your kid is dodging bullets just to get on the school bus. My husband buys me furs and cars for Christmas, your husband, who loves you no less, buys you a bottle of perfume. Since you are my friend, I want to share with you the happy moments as well as the sad, so each time my hubby does something extra special for me I want to tell you. We take trips to Paris and the Bahamas; you take trips to the Smokey Mountains. How do you feel? Do you talk bad about me because you think I'm bragging? Should I not tell you about my happy moments because you and your hubby don't have the resources to express yourself with lavish gifts? Can we really be friends? I've never been rich, but we have been quite comfortable so I must say this. The test of prosperity is a far greater test than the test of poverty. And if you have the pleasure of experiencing both, in the same lifetime, you will know the joy of true friendship. Once you have gone full circle, it's only your true friends that are left when the dust settles. To my true friends…I love you and appreciate you more than you'll ever know. You are a true gift of God. I won't name names because you know who you are.

Saturday, October 19, 2002 2:22 pm

*I*t's a rainy Saturday afternoon, and Taylor's finally down for her afternoon nap. I'm glad my hubby has been taking care of her today, I needed the break. I think I want to talk about relationships today. The quest to find your soul mate or for your soul mate to find you, whatever the case may be is a somewhat daunting task. Many people believe that if you ever have hard times, or moments when you feel like walking out the door and never coming back, that you must not be with your soulmate. That's not always the case. The thing that people don't understand is that only you and God know if someone is your soul mate or not. No one else has the right to make that judgement. And the funny thing about God is, he actually wants you talk to him about if a person is your soul mate, and after you finish talking, take the time to listen. He may not say anything, but there's so much handwriting on the wall you can't deny it one way or the other. Some people, especially women, want to get married so badly, that they could care less if a person is their soul mate. If he has a job and walks upright, that's all the criteria they need to make their decision. Some people think they can eventually change a person into what they want; all they have to do is get them down the aisle first. It ain't gonna happen cap'ain. The person you marry is the person you got for life, unless they are your soul mate.

If they're your soul mate a miraculous phenomenon happens. God uses you to tweak them, and them to tweak you, and circumstances and hardships to tweak both of you at the same time. As you grow and mature and are tweaked together, an unstoppable, undeniable, unshakable alliance is created. When that happens you will let no thing or no one (not even yourself) destroy what God has created. It's amazing. That's what marriage is supposed to be. It's not this Hollywood-pie-in-the-sky nor is it the depths of hell, it's somewhere in between, and if you do it right, your good days will outweigh your bad. What more could you ask for? This is dedicated to my soul mate, my hubby, and my friend...and the Awesome God that tweaks us.

Sunday, October 20, 2002 5:12 PM

🦋

*I*t's another lazy Sunday afternoon and today is a good day. I got up and went to church this morning while my hubby watched the baby. It was a really good sermon. I feel very, very grateful to be in great health, with no aches and no pains! That's an inside joke. About 7 years ago, one of my baby-cousins was diagnosed with a Wilm's tumor. She was about 3 years old at the time. After several months of chemo and radiation, I took her and a few of my other baby cousins out for ice cream and the park. I drove past the Hospital where she went for her daily "treatments." The girls were in the backseat giggling and having fun and just being kids. As we passed the hospital my little cousin with the most adult voice I had heard up to that point shouted, "I don't have to go back to the hospital no more, 'cause I don't have no aches and no pains!" As she said this she waved her little finger back and forth, it was the cutest thing you'd ever want to see. Then they continued with their miniature conversation. I was in the front seat laughing and crying quietly to myself. Look at that little butterfly, I was so proud of her! She's now 10 years old and a 7-year cancer survivor. It's amazing to see a <u>child</u> with the strength to fight one of the most debilitating diseases known in our time. The thing that people don't understand about cancer and any other chronic disease, is that you have to fight every day. You have to fight the desire to give up on life when things aren't going well. You have to fight the negative thoughts. You have to fight the fear that you could have passed a defective gene down to your offspring. You have to fight...you have to fight. YOU HAVE TO FIGHT! And when you get tired of fighting, you'd better have a GOD to call on to fight for you until you get your second wind...because from here on out you have to fight, for now and the rest of your life. The great thing about all this is that I have always loved a good fight.

Monday, October 21, 2002 7:11 PM

This day will go unrecorded.

Wednesday, October 23, 2002 8:02 PM

🦋

y baby is 10 months old today and she took her first steps at about 5:00 this evening. I'm so excited and so proud of her. I'm glad my hubby and I were able to witness this for ourselves because, I promise you, if I had to hear this from some babysitter, I would be seething mad right now. It was the cutest thing. She held on to the couch, then she let go, with her chubby feet, moving one in from of the other for about three steps. The funny thing is the more we clapped for her, the more she wanted to do it. I told my hubby we have to get this on tape. I was so happy I cried a little. It's amazing to see her grow up before my very eyes. Oh, by the way, I donated all my maternity and "fat" clothes to the YWCA. I had some really cute stuff, but I don't think I'm having any more children and even if I do, someone could use those things right now. Otherwise they'll just sit in my closet collecting dust. You know, we're really living in scary times. That "Maryland Sniper" is going around killing and shooting people by the handfuls, and then they released the news that he's threatening children. Crazy, crazy, crazy. This person is crazy with a twist of lemon. I pray for the families that have lost their loved ones. We are really living in crazy times. I actually went to get my wig fixed today. It's been too long. When I came home Taylor kept staring at me like, I was some new person; I certainly feel like one. I must look nice because Mork said; "oh…your hair looks nice." Or he'll wait until the hairdo has run its course and say, "I really liked your hair a week ago." Men are weird. I've come to that conclusion.

Thursday, October 24, 2002 9:02 AM

🦋

Supposedly they caught the "Maryland Sniper" today. Over the past few weeks, I've been praying, "…please don't let him be black." Is that a bad thing to say? I'm just thinking, all we need is another reason to be racially pro-filed, or to have more of our teenagers beat to a bloody pulp simply because they "fit the profile" of an offender. And of course to my surprise and dismay, the two suspects are black. They're trying to say that they're not white or black but Jamaican, but when I saw their pictures, they looked black to me. I hope they've really caught the sniper and they're not just using these guys as a decoy to appease the public. I pray to God that they have the right guys, and that justice is served. God, please don't let another innocent man get the electric chair. It makes me very sad to think about it. I hope they've caught the right people. I was talking to my hubby today, asking if he thought we were living on Fantasy Island. I'm trying to write my book, he's trying to get his music thing going and neither of us have jobs. We've been looking like crazy for him a job, but the competition is fierce right now because of the economy. Thanks George! They tell him he's overqualified for just about everything he goes for, and since that is the case, no employer wants to take him on for fear he'll leave. I'm really at a loss as to what to do. Man, even though I want to be home with Taylor, I even started looking for a contract position just to tie us over. It's really a rough time for us right now. We aren't starving and we haven't lost anything, but I wish things would turn around for us soon. My Dad always says, "What doesn't kill you makes you strong." Well, I don't know if I can handle any more strength!

Friday, October 25, 2002 7:28 PM

*I*t's Friday night and I feel good. I feel better physically than I've felt in a long time. And, I must say, I look good too. Thanks God, for that freebie, I appreciate it. It's a bad situation when things are going bad and you look bad too. But I have to say, my face has a certain glow to it that I'm very thankful for. I e-mailed some of my family and friends to tell them Taylor was walking, I am so pumped about that. My little baby is walking! It is so amazing to think that just a few months ago she would just lay there and blow spit bubbles. Now she's standing, walking, feeding herself, and trying to talk. It's really amazing. I know I keep using that word over and over, but that's the best description I can come up with. I remember back in the day, before I had Taylor, people would tell me about their kids starting to walk. I would say something like, "get out of here. Are you serious?" You know, the canned responses you give when something is obviously more of a big deal to someone else than it is to you. Now that I have experienced the joy of seeing my first child walk on her own for the first time, I finally understand what all the hoopla is about. It's a Mommy-Thing. I feel really grateful to be living the life I'm living. I have a good hubby, a beautiful daughter and a great extended family. That's worth so much more than money. Now don't get me wrong, money is important...but there is lot of things worth so much more. Well. I'm going to end on that note because the Lakers and Kings are about to play. See you tomorrow, God willing.

Saturday, October 26, 2002 10:22 AM

🦋

*I*t's Saturday morning and I still didn't get enough sleep. Taylor whined for a good part of the night because she wanted to sleep in our bed. Her routine works like this. She stays in our bed until she falls asleep, I mean really asleep, and we put her in her bed. If she wakes up during the night, which happens every once and a while, she comes back to our bed until she falls asleep. Our bed is not that big, so hubby and I are usually sleep-depraved by morning. She sleeps like a baby, as she should, and we walk around all day like zombies. Well last night hubby decides that she has to learn to sleep in her own bed, so you know how that went. I was pretty upset because I just wanted her to be quiet and go to sleep so I could sleep. So she goes through a lot of drama until he finally gets her to fall asleep and she sleeps in her own bed all night. He tells me later that he knows how to deal with her drama because that's how he was when he was a kid. That's obviously some defective gene he passed on to our child. Just kidding, Taylor, when you learn how to read and you see this line, I'm only kidding. There's nothing defective about you. I was thinking about my parents early this morning and last night. Neither of them came from the best possible situations, but they somehow stuck it out long enough to bring 2 of their 6 children to adulthood, before splitting up. I have the utmost respect for both of them in different ways. They did the best they could with the tools given to them. We all grew up to be good, honest people and 4 of us have graduated college. In fact my big sister was the first in our family to receive her Masters Degree. My parents did a heck of a job. When I look at some of the things my peers have experienced during their childhood, at the hand of their parents, I thank God for a "normal" family. It's my job to pick up the baton where my parents left off, and take parenthood to the next level. I want to be the best mother I can be. I really think, I'm done having children. I want to be able to give Taylor my all and still have something left for myself. I don't know if I can do that if I have another child. It's really not on my list of things to do. Maybe I'll feel differently later but I really doubt it. And you know what…I don't care what anybody thinks, with all the torture my body has been through, I will not have a child without my mind and my body's consent. It just doesn't make good sense. Several people have told me, "Oh, you need to have a least one more." Or they'll say, "You've got to have a little boy." Says who! First of all, none of these people have to carry the child in their scar-tissued uterus. Nor do they have to change a diaper or wake up for one 3 o'clock feeding. Let's not even get into clothing and feeding the child for the next 18 + years. Then there's the issue of having a boy. You know, when I was pregnant I would have been just as happy to have a boy as I was to have girl. It was just the fact that I really wanted a healthy child. But somehow, in our archaic society, you still have to have a boy. Either they say, "Have a boy for your husband." Or they say, "Taylor needs a brother." The only thing Taylor needs is the two loving parents she has, and God. I really get angry about that. As if, I can wave some magic 8-ball across my stomach and a baby boy will appear instead of a girl. And if anybody thinks I'm going to let them take some embryos and spin them around in a centrifuge and put back only the ones that show up with a Y-chromosome, they are mad! I mean mad-cow, Mad-Hatter mad.

Monday, October 28, 2002 4:35 P.M.

❦

I know we didn't talk yesterday…but there's a very good reason. I lost my mind yesterday! I'm joking but I'm not. Yesterday was one of the worst days I've had in a long time. It was just an overwhelming day. There wasn't anything in particular that happened it was just one of those days when you're tired of looking on the bright-side of everything. You're tired of saying to yourself, "Things are going to get better real soon." Simply put, you come to the end of your hope. Yesterday I was all hoped out. I was fed up with hoping the ideal job would come through for my hubby. I was fed up with hoping that his music career would take off for him. I was fed up with hoping that life, motherhood, and womanhood would one day get easier. I can't ever remember being as emotionally, mentally, physically, socially and spiritually tired as I was yesterday. So you see that was not a good day for us to talk. I just cried, screamed, threw clothes, and fussed while my hubby was playing with Taylor in the next room. When I was finished with my tantrum, I just asked God to help me and I fell asleep. He had to have touched me during my nap because when I woke up, I felt like a new person. I've decided that I am going to slowly give up my "control-freak" position, because trying to control things that are outside of my control is not only insane, it's killing me. And trust me, if I wanted to die, I would have gave in 11 years ago when the "Big C" first came knocking on my campus apartment door. I'm going to learn to let go, with God's help, because I'm so tired I can't see straight. Today, however, is a much better day.

Tuesday, October 29, 2002 9:39 AM

🦋

Today I have my 6-month appointment with the oncologist. They usually take my blood, check for lumps, check my breathing, etc., etc. I used to be afraid, each time I had one of these appointments, because experience had taught me to expect the worse. I'm not afraid today, because I'm just trusting God to take care of me. I'm really upset with myself, because my plan was to have lost more weight by this time, but you know how that goes. I ate a full course meal at about 10:00 PM, something I normally don't do. Taylor woke up bright-eyed and bushy-tailed this morning, so did hubby. I guess I'll go now and tell you how the appointment went. See Ya!

4:58 PM

All went well at my Doctor's appointment. Thank God for that.

Wednesday, October 30, 2002 12:40 PM

❦

O k, I'm really grossed out. I just visited one of my favorite fast food joints, and I was just about to take the second bite of my delicious cheeseburger, only to discover something was caught on my tooth. "It must be an onion," I said trying to reassure myself. But it wasn't. I'm trying to suppress my desire to upchuck just <u>telling</u> this story. It was a long blond hair. And I'm not a blond! I gagged, then I spit out the unchewed bite I still had in my mouth. I guess I'm fortunate…I could have found something far worse. I feel like cooks, did it on purpose. I don't know why, because I go out of my way not to upset anyone while they're preparing, serving, or handling my food. In fact, if I think someone has something against me, I do not eat the food they cook. Ma said, "…you can't eat everybody's food." I brought a couple of sandwiches back for hubby, but told him I was taking mine back to get my money back, due to the hair. He said, "…it happens." As if I had said I found an extra pickle on my burger or something. I asked if he still wanted his sandwiches. He said, "Yep." I have a true caveman on my hands. In my opinion, nothing short of a swarm of cockroaches, that can gross me out more than finding hair in my food, and he say, "it happens." Go figure. Men are from the Stone Age; Women are from Venus… I'm getting more and more excited about my trip to NY. The hustle and bustle will seem like heaven compared to the landfill of doody diapers I've changed over the past 10 months. It's all very exciting. No husbands, no babies, no doo doo, no bill collectors to avert; it will just be my big sis and me on the town.

Friday, November 1, 2002 8:56 AM

It's amazing this year is almost over...where did the time go. I went back to my routine of not eating after 7:30 PM. So far its working great I've lost 4 lbs in just two days and I'm eating everything I want within reason. I finally got a good night's rest. Taylor kept me up Wednesday night and I was so bushed I forgot to do anything. Hence, we haven't talked since Wednesday. Taylor's going through this phase that she doesn't want to sleep in her own bed, so Wednesday night I tried to sleep with her on the couch in the den. This child tossed and turned and kicked until about 7:00 am the next morning. That's when I finally got to get a couple hours of sleep then she woke up bright-eyed and bushy-tailed. Speaking of which, she's up now. Last night her Dad had her so I could get some sleep; I wonder if he got any sleep last night? Oh, by the way, I don't know if I'm a glutton for punishment but I'm think of working as a nursery attendant at a nearby church. It doesn't pay much of anything, it's really a labor of love...so why am I doing this? I don't love strangers' children. Those are the kids that kick you in the shin and tell their parents you were mean to them. I thought it would be a good way to get Taylor to interact with other kids her age without paying "baby gym" prices. It sounds less and less like a good idea now. I'm supposed to be there at 10:00 AM to fill out the application, then they I have to stop by the police station to pick up my criminal record, or the lack thereof in my case. Then they have to check my references. You know I think it's important that all these checks be done to insure the safety of all children, it's just now, that I've thought it through, do I want to go through all of this for a few bucks a week. I mean they only need me for 6-8 hours per week. To make matters worse, they want me to work on Sunday mornings. I know me…if I chase toddlers, early Sunday morning, it's going to be too easy for me not to go to church when it's time to leave. And this church is right around the corner from my house and my church is all the way across town. It would be too easy, to just round the corner and come home after work. Nice try, Devil…we need money but I'm not missing church!

Saturday, November 2, 2002 10:10 AM

*W*ell last night hubby got a lead on a job from someone
he used to work with, so we'll see how that goes. I
ain't holding my breath because I have no idea what God's
will is concerning this position so as always it's a wait and
see type of deal. You know I was thinking the other day
about the day Taylor was born. The night before, I starting
having contractions but there was no rhyme or reason to the
frequency. That night hubby was putting the crib together
while I got the rest of my things packed for the hospital
stay. I told him right before I went to bed, "…oh I'll probably have the baby tomorrow." He said, "What?" Then I
repeated what I had said. He said ok, like he didn't believe
me. I got up about 10:00 AM the next morning to shower,
and to finish getting the last minute things in order. Then I
told him to get ready, because by that time my contractions
were about 5 minutes apart. He said, "What?!" So I repeated
myself. I don't hold it against him, it's our first child and
he didn't know what to do or what to expect. Well he got
ready and he was driving me to the hospital. The contractions were starting to be a little more intense, but I wasn't
in any real pain. Hubby started getting scared, asking me
every time I paused from talking, if I was ok. I told him, I
was ok and that he should stop and get him something to
eat, because once we got to the hospital, he wouldn't be able

to leave for a while. He asked me if I was crazy, and said he wasn't stopping for any food. I said, "Well at least stop for gas, the tank is about on E." He didn't stop for gas either he just continued to drive me to the hospital. When we got there, it was about 1:30PM…hold on, we'll continue this later, it's time for Taylor's breakfast.

4:17 PM

Okay, back to my story. When we got to the hospital the nurse said they didn't see any contractions on the monitor, but the contractions were in my back and the monitor is only designed to pick up contractions in the front. So they figured it was all in my mind or Braxton-Hicks, and were about to send me home. But hubby went out of the room, talked to somebody and raised some sand, telling them that if I say I'm having contractions then I must be. I don't know what else he said, but they were just taking orders from my doctor, who was, I'm imagining, chilling in her cozy, little million-dollar home. Oh, and this was on a Sunday, two days before Christmas. So she was probably decking the halls by now. Since my hubby refused to take me back home they decided to run an IV drip that had water and electrolytes and such, because they figured I was just dehydrated. I just started praying because I have a friend who had a similar experience and it turned out to be a horrible ordeal for her. So as they IV started dripping, instead of my contractions dying down, as they expected, they started to get more intense, and by the grace of God, moved to the front were the monitor could pick them up! The contractions were starting to be about a minute apart, and although I don't remember feeling any pain at all, they did take my breath. The nurse finally saw one on the monitor and it was huge. I guess they felt that because I wasn't screaming, I must not be about to have a baby. But whether they liked it or not, Taylor was coming. They started getting me prepped for the scheduled C-section and then my doctor showed up as if appearing from thin air. So it was about 5:00 PM at this point and they were putting me in surgery garb, and I realized, my hubby had not returned from grabbing a sandwich from the hospital cafeteria. So he had no clue the baby was going to be there in a matter of minutes. I had him paged and he still had not showed up. I started to panic, thinking, of all the things I've been through, if this man misses the birth of our first child, I'll have a divorce lawyer stand in for him. Everybody was waiting then he finally showed up. He was in the bathroom, doing number 2. I told him, "Get your scrubs on, they're about to take the baby." "Now?" he said. "Yes, now!" He looked as if I slapped him then slowly started to get dressed. The nurse came in to hurry him along then they whisked me away. At 5:31 PM on Sunday, December 23, 2001, I gave birth to a beautiful, bubbly, bouncing baby girl. She weighed 8 lbs and 3 oz and according to my hubby and the nurses, she came out fighting. As I heard her scream I just cried and cried, because it had been such a long journey to get her here safe and sound. Then I thought, oh my Lord…I have a baby!

Today is a great day. But it didn't start out that way. It was another one of those days were I was having a pity party because I really expected to be rich at this stage in my life. Don't ask me why, but I remember growing up thinking, I'm going to be rich one day. No, I'm not a great singer; no I don't have a jump-shot; and I haven't discovered a cure for cancer. I just equated the fact that I was smart as a child to being rich as an adult. Boy was I wrong. Some of the dumbest people known to man, are as rich as they are dumb. I'm not going to name any, because you may know a few of them. Then I think about the great thinkers of our time. None of them were rich; most of them didn't even die rich. It's amazing. Our society rewards talent with money, and intellect with ostracism. I remember when I was a kid, they called me brainy-smurf, so I would literally hold back in class, so that I wouldn't be labeled as the teacher's pet, or my favorite nick-name, "Brainiac." Now, don't get me wrong, there were a lot of kids that were just as smart, and smarter than I. But there were not trying to be accepted by the "cool" kids like I was. Finally when I was in 9th grade I gave up. I gave up trying to "dumb it down" for my friends (and I use the term loosely). I started answering questions I knew in class. I started expressing my disappointment to others when I got a "B" and not an "A." I sat far away from the people who would distract me while I was trying to take notes or listen in class. I started to stand up and be me. By the time I was in 11th grade I was named Who's Who Among American High School Students, Governor's Scholar, and received 3 scholarships that offered me a full ride to college. Then, I was invited to apply to Stanford University. All of those things were great accomplishments for a 17-year-old. But now I'm almost 33 years old, educated, relatively cultured, and darn near a cornucopia of useless facts. So what do I do with my knowledge? I play Jeopardy online, hoping one day I'll get up the nerve and to go try out for the television version. Since I know now that it is my destiny to triumph magnificently on that show!

Monday, November 4, 2002 1:50 PM

W e're another day closer to my trip to NY. I am so excited!!! Away from babies and husbands for 48 whole hours, three cheers, hip hip hooray! Hip hip Hooray! I've already started packing. I just need to get my toiletries together and then we're off! Yaaaaaaa! I guessed you can tell I'm amped about my trip. It's been a long time coming. I'm not going to talk about the job situation or situations, because I don't want you to bring me down. God will supply all of my need according to his riches in glory. I just have to learn to believe that as much as I believe, "with his stripes, I am healed." It's been a long journey. I guess I don't have much else to say. We'll talk again tomorrow.

10:22 PM

I got a call earlier today from my Uncle Mike. I mean, he is by far one of my favorite uncles of all time. In fact when we were little kids, he used to quiz us. "Who's your favorite uncle?" And we'd say, "Uncle Mike." Then he'd give us a kiss, and sometimes a dollar bill and walk away smiling. Well, today he called me to tell me he has 90% blockage to one of the main arteries of his heart. He gave me more details but, it seems like such a bad dream that the specifics are a little hazy. The bottom line is that he has to have a quadruple-by-pass on this coming Friday and he told me that he's made his peace with God and that if he doesn't come out of it, he wants me to know that he loves me. You have no idea how hard this for me. Uncle Mike told me that he's already told my aunt, his children and staff at the church. He's a pastor of a large congregation and one of the few godly men left on this earth. He's telling our extended family tomorrow. I told him I loved him more than he would ever know and that I would be praying. Then I reminded him of how God has kept me alive. Twelve years and two bouts of cancer later, I'm still here by the grace of God. I also told him about my scripture that I quote constantly. "He was wounded for my transgressions, he was bruised for my iniquities, the chastisement of my peace was upon him and with his stripes I am healed." I told him that I'm living on the words of God. He told me that he wanted me to give my testimony when I come back in town and that he was going to start quoting that scripture also. I also told him about how that scripture got me through even as a child with asthma, and that once I began quoting that scripture, I never had another asthma attack. He was encouraged. It felt good to encourage my uncle, since he has always encouraged me, even in my darkest hours. I really love him. This day is dedicated to my uncle, Dr. Michael E. Ford Sr. He is truly a great man of God.

Tuesday, November 5, 2002 3:43 PM

🦋

*H*ubby and I took Taylor with us to vote today. She was so fascinated by the lights hanging in the ceiling of the gymnasium that was our designated polling place. I thought about voting straight-party ticket, but then I decided to go with the candidates I believed would be least likely to support a war. Call it the flower-child in me but I don't want my daughter growing up in the midst of a war. For the first time in my life I feel the U.S. is vulnerable to a war on our "turf." It used to seem so far-fetched, but since 9/11, I think we as Americans realize that there are a lot of people in this world that hate us. Some hate us for good reasons and others, for not-so-good reasons. In my opinion, the bottom-line is we need to focus on foreign and domestic terrorism and leave Sadaam alone. These are really troubling times. Last night I had a hard time sleeping. I guess I had my Uncle's surgery on my mind. Then when I finally thought I'd be able to doze off, hubby started snoring; it wasn't really loud, but just loud enough to keep me from going to sleep. I want to call my sister and tell her about my uncle but part of me feels like I should wait till I get to NY. Then again, if something goes wrong, she would have never known he was even going in for surgery and that would be horrible. So I guess I'll call her tonight and tell her. I'm going to wait a little while to give myself a chance to come up with the right terminology to describe the situation. I want her to know the seriousness of the circumstances, but I don't want to upset her real bad and not be there to comfort her. Who am I kidding? I'm not the greatest comforter, when it comes to my big sis. I mean she's my Big Sis, so it feels awkward to have to comfort her if she cries or something. Well, I'll do my best if it comes to that. I know she would do it for me.

Wednesday, November 6, 2002 1:10 PM

It's another day. I had to erase what I wrote earlier because it just wasn't nice. I feel better now.

T'm going to take Taylor with me to get my hair done today. This should be an adventure. Well, when I got my hair braided she did pretty well, considering it was a 9-hour ordeal. This is simply a wash and blow-dry, so it should be ok. I know that's boring conversation so let's change the subject. I talked to Ma the other night, she was really worried about my uncle, and I can understand; he's her baby brother for crying out loud. Oh by the way when I talked to my big sis the other day to tell her about my uncle's surgery, she handled it very well. And I found out he's having a quadruple by-pass and not a triple by-pass. I'm just praying that all goes well and that God will give him a speedy recovery. I'm also going to pray that his congregation leave him alone and let him recuperate. He's going to be flat on his back for 6-8 weeks. It's really a scary ordeal; my uncle is just turning 50 years old. Well, I jump on the plane to go to NY tomorrow. Have I told you how amped I am? Well, I AM AMPED!!!!

10:08 PM

It's me again. I'm starting to have mixed feelings about leaving Taylor. I mean, I've never been away from her longer that 12 hours and that's when my brother and his girlfriend watched her overnight when I went home to visit last August. Men don't always have the patience that women have when it comes to their children. But the patience we have acquired didn't come overnight. I'll be gone for only 52 hours so, I'm sure they'll be fine. Hubby was teasing saying he was going to find somebody to watch her while I'm gone. He's just yanking my chain because he is just as particular about who she's around as I am. For some strange reason, it's like he wants me to worry, like deep down he's jealous that I'm going to be out and about in NY, having fun, while he's here with the baby. I have one thing to say about that. WELCOME TO MY WORLD! I'm not going to worry about anything. I'm going to put it all in God hands like I do any other time. There's only so much I can do. I can't be at 5 places at once, I can't please everybody all the time, nor am I going to try. I've learned the hard way that no matter how many people need me, or how many people I think need me, I need me more than any of them. So I'm going to make sure I do everything in my power to see about me first. Yes, that means if I take a 2 day hiatus from wifery and motherhood, its for my own good as well as the good of my family. I've learned that the worse thing I can do for my relationships is to let myself get burned out. So, I no longer do. Everybody needs a break every once and a while. And for those couples who have never spent a night apart, God bless you. That's all I have to say about that. My Uncle has his surgery early tomorrow morning. I've been praying for him everyday. Surgery is a scary thing. I've had 8, so I'm not just whistling Dixie as they say. The night before you try to get a good night sleep but it's almost impossible because you're on pins and needles about how the surgery will go, and what they will find when the open you up, etc., etc. But I've learned to just tell myself to "prepare for the best sleep you've ever had in your life." And it is. You don't remember anything, you don't dream. They tell you to start counting backwards, then everything goes white. Then you wake right back up like "Hey they forgot to put me to sleep!" Then you realize that the surgery is over and you've been asleep or "under" for an hour. It's an amazing thing. Scientists say having general anesthesia is the closest you'll ever get to death without actually dying. Lord…just let my Uncle be ok…

Friday, November 8, 2002 8:49 AM

A lot of things are going on today. My uncle is in surgery even as we speak. I pray that all goes well. Hubby has an interview for a contract position today at 11:00 AM. I leave for NY today. I automatically woke up today at 6:24 AM. My uncle's surgery started at 6:30 AM, my time. I prayed for him until I got sleepy again and then fell asleep. I'm pretty worried. Ma said she would give me a call when the surgery is over to give me his status. I don't have much else to say.

Monday, November 11, 2002 1:55 AM

T'm back from NY and I had a great time!

Wednesday, November 13, 2002 7:55 AM

I feel so refreshed! I had a nice little two-day break and I literally feel like a new woman. It was good to see family that I hadn't seen in a while and it was also good to chill out with my sister, just me and her. She lives in a nice neighborhood in Brooklyn. Her apartment is surrounded by bookstores, little bohemian shops, and quaint little cafés. We had a great time. It was nice just to get out and about in the city. I had a blast!

Thursday, November 14, 2002 8:31 AM

Taylor decided not to go to sleep until about 1:00 AM this morning. Then she wakes up a 7:30 AM like she has to go into the office today or something. I don't know where she gets the energy because I am exhausted. I don't know if I have jet-lag or what but I am really, really tired.

Friday, November 15, 2002 10:09 AM

W ell hubby had an 2nd interview today. He found out late this afternoon that he didn't get the position and no one would tell him why when he asked. I told him not to worry; things will turn around at some point. I guess I don't have much else to say. Oh yes I do…So far my uncle is doing great. Thank God for that. That's worth more than money.

Sunday November 17, 2002 6:47 PM

❦

I guess my muse has left me. I have nothing to write about. I feel that if I have to write about my feelings of gloom and doom, I'd better not write at all. I feel like my parents. In the early years they raised us on a wing and a prayer financially speaking. They were too poor to have enough, but not poor enough to get assistance. I think we're worse off than they were because right now I think we qualify, for just about any assistance there is out there because we literally have no income. I've told my family this once or twice, but I don't think they get the gist because I'm not making it a big deal. And hubby was right, money, or the lack thereof does affect a relationship. You don't even have the time or the energy to think about that pie-in-the-sky love life you once had, because you're too busy worrying about bills. I have to be honest and come clean. There are enemies out there that would love to gloat over, our "hard times." Man, there might even be some enemies disguised as friends that would want to gloat over our financial misfortune. So I tell as few people as possible. I don't want to give them the satisfaction of laughing at my calamity. I have to give hubby props, because he will tell anybody, anytime, anywhere that we are struggling. But he's never been poor like I have. I know what it's like to be made fun of because you wear the latest styles from DAV's. And their latest style was two decades ago. I remember being ashamed to tell my schoolmates that I lived on the West End, because that side of town was immediately associated with poverty, crime and drugs. I've been on the wrong side of money most of my life, so you think I would get used to it. But I refuse. I will not be poor all my life. I have to say, it really hurts to be poor most of your life, struggle through college which is a whole different level of poverty, then make it out of college, get married to an educated man and you and he both become professionals, making money your parents could only dream of making, then after 4 years, it all gets snatched away. Or you give it away, unknowingly, whatever the case may be. However you lost it, is just as painful. The ache of poverty literally makes me sick to my stomach, so I have to call on God to help me. A wise man once told me that the test of prosperity is a far greater test than the test of poverty. We'll see old man, we'll see.

🦋

I'm really not in the mood for the cutesy way I've been writing before. I just don't feel cutesy at all. Don't misunderstand, I still feel cute, aesthetically speaking, but that bubble gum pie in the sky cutesy me is gone. The full fledge woman of turmoil, struggle, and survival has submerged. I'm tired of acting like everything is ok; everything is not ok! It will be okay, one day, some day, but I don't know when that day is so, I have to take it one day at a time. I think I picked up some bug from somewhere because I feel lousy. My throat is killing me. Well, I'm exaggerating, as long as I don't have to swallow, it's bearable. But who wants to hold their saliva in their mouth all day. It just doesn't work well when holding a conversation with someone. I go to the food stamp office on Wednesday of this week, and I'm actually excited about it. The excitement comes in when I think about the fact that I can continue to feed my child nourishing meals. I'm definitely hyped about that. Otherwise, the actual going to the food stamp office is far less thrilling. It's humiliating and to see the look on the Case Worker's face when they see how much money you used to make, it gives you mixed emotions because you don't know if they're going to give you a hard time, or feel sorry for you or treat you like trash. It's a toss-up. I've determined in my heart that I'm going to chronicle the events of my life until things turn around for us. And I mean in a big way. So if it takes 3 months, a year, or 10 years so be it. We'll either have a pamphlet on our hands or a duplicate of <u>War and Peace</u> up in this piece! Either way I hope to help and/or inspire somebody out there. Because at some point in your life, you will be able to identify with me because life doesn't get any easier, you just learn to hand more of it over to God, you know, to keep you from losing your mind. I think writing is very good for me because I really don't like telling people my problems. I just think when you're verbally wallowing in your own self-pity, you're usually the last person to get invited to someone else's celebration. And I do love to celebrate other people's good fortune. Heck, I love to celebrate my own good fortune!

Wednesday, November 20, 2002 9:45 AM

esterday was a bad day...I mean a really bad day. I can't even begin to tell you how bad it was; it was just bad. Thank God for the "magic" he performs in our lives to turn confusion and chaos into calm and tranquility. I mean it's like after a horrendous storm, the trees are falling down, the thunder sounds like it splitting the sky in two, then the storm passes, the sun is shining and the birds are chirping like, "storm, what storm?" That's how it was today, the calm after the storm. But there is some debris lying around here and there that needs to be picked up, and there were a few branches that fell in your yard, but nothing major. That is how today was. Thank God for divine intervention, our lives would be a mess without it. I went in for an interview today. We really need the money, but I told God and I meant it, that if it is in his divine will for me to get that particular job I will, and if it's not, I am not going to cry about it or even be disappointed. I'm just going to say Amen. The reason I've had this epiphany is this. All my life, I've begged God for things I felt like I just couldn't do without. Then when I get them it's like, why in the name of all that is holy, did I beg for something that has caused me so much stress and heartache that I literally felt like I was losing my mind. I can't begin to tell you about the jobs I begged God for, and then when I got them I was like, "Oh my God what have I

63

gotten myself into." Some people may think it's being ungrateful. God knows I'm grateful for everything he has given me and everything he has enabled me to do. I can only speak for myself, but I think God is showing me to let him be in charge because nobody knows the future like he does. It's a life-lesson. Stop begging God for stuff and pray his will. Now I don't have a problem praying for things like health for myself and my family, financial security, debts paid off, but I afterward I put in the disclaimer. "Lord, I ask this is Jesus name, if it be according to your perfect will. And I mean I do this with everything now. I have made too many messes in life that God has had to come back and clean up, just so I can live a healthy, happy life. It's amazing, his mess-fixing ability, it's also very humbling. I want to talk about me a little. I think I touched on it a little and God knows it's been my daily prayer of late. I'm so tired of caring about what people think. I have a phobia that people will judge me, and they probably are, but I'm asking God to help me not to care. I care way too much about what people think and it has been very debilitating to my life. All I can say is me and God are working on it. He has to do the big stuff because I have no idea where to begin. I mean I really have no idea. My childhood was happy for the most part, but I was such a sensitive soul, that I can probably remember every derogatory statement someone said to or about me. I remember when I was about 8 years old and in the 3rd grade. I was at school and I had to go to the little girl's room so of course, my teacher let me go. When I got in the stall the other two stalls to the right and the left of me was occupied by two 5th graders. They were talking to each other back and forth as girls will do while using the facilities. Then one of them asked the other who was in the middle stall, and of course it was me. I was extremely shy so I didn't say anything at first, then they asked again, so I identified myself. Then I heard the words that would haunt me for the rest of my life. "Oh that's that girl who wears those ugly clothes -her mother must not care about her." I feel so silly, because the thought of those words, even now makes my eyes well up, but as I told you before I was and still am a sensitive soul. I was crushed. It wasn't so much what they said, because I knew my mother loved me dearly, it was the fact these two people that I had never did or said anything against could be so mean and cruel to me for no reason. I ran into one of the girls since we've been adults, she had no clue that she left such an indelible mark on my psyche, and of course I never mentioned it. I found out from talking to her that she was sent to boarding school after leaving our elementary school. She also has a chronic case of diabetes, where she passes out and goes into comas on a dime. I pray for her every time I think about her, nobody should have to suffer that way. Well we'll talk about whether I got the job or not tomorrow…if no more storms blow through.

𝒯aylor is 11 months old today and into everything this morning. I think I'm going to go ahead and wean her off formula over the next several days and start giving her whole milk. I didn't get the job that we talked about the other day but there are a couple of interviews that are scheduled for next week so I should come up with something. Hubby is just being offered crappy weekend jobs but he takes them because we need the money. The job market is really ugly right now. People like me and hubby who used to get great jobs on a dime are settling for entry level temp work just to stay afloat. It's definitely a humbling experience. Oh, by the way. Something extraordinary happened yesterday. I don't know if I told you but for the last 3 ½ years hubby has been working on getting his music out. That was the whole purpose of him starting his business back in 1999. Well, yesterday he received a letter from the leading entertainment law firm, saying that they thought his music production ability was very good and that they would like to work with him on some level. That letter is definitely a step in the right direction. It happened like this. I was driving to the store and decided before I left our neighborhood to stop by our mailbox. It one of those compartmentalized community mailboxes. I opened our box and retrieved the goo-goobs of bills and junk mail that we receive on the daily. I sifted through everything and saw a letter from an attorney's office in New York. My first thought was, "ok who's trying to sue us." But I went ahead and opened it. The letter read, as I said before, that the firm thought the music on hubby's demo was "very good" and that they "would like to work with him on some level." That was enough for me because I know how hubby has been fighting to get a break on his music, since that is his first love. I left the car parked at the mailbox, with nothing in my hand but the letter and ran down the street back to our townhouse. I opened the door, completely out of breath and went into the kitchen where hubby and Taylor were. I said, "Here, read this." Hubby looked a little scared and asked what it was. I was trying to tell him but I'm sure I was speaking so incoherently he couldn't make heads or tails of what I was saying. So I said, "Just read it." And he did. And his face lit up. I asked him was I misinterpreting the letter or was it really good news like I thought. He said, "No, this is good news." Then I saw it. Something I haven't seen in months. His face completely lit up. "Come give me hug." he said. I did, congratulated him, then I left to go to the grocery to try to make a dollar out of 15 cents. I know I had less than 60 dollars to buy groceries for hubby myself and Taylor to last until the next time we get some money. Earlier this week I had even went to apply for food stamps. Things are just that bad. They said we didn't qualify because of some red-tape garbage, but told me to reapply in December. In the mean time they handed me a coupon to receive a free turkey basket from a local church. At first I thought to myself, I'm not going to get any turkey basket...things aren't that bad. But yesterday I realized that they actually are that bad, so I swallowed a mouthful of pride and drove to the church to pick up our Thanksgiving basket. I also got a free turkey from the grocery for making a purchase over $50. So hubby and I should be able to eat off this for at least a couple of weeks. I purchased quite a bit of baby finger food for Taylor so she'll be eating better than her mom and dad. I don't mind, because her health and welfare always comes first. This has been a very educational week. I hope my experience will help somebody else someday.

I have to be honest; I hate adversity. It seems to rear its ugly head in every aspect of my life. Now I could take the spiritual approach and say, "it will all work out for my good." And I know eventually it will, but the actual going through the adversity part is not fun, not at all. I may be starting a new job tomorrow that I really don't want. Let me rephrase that. I want the part of the job that involves, receiving money, but the actual job part, I don't know. It's a nickel and dime job, making $12/hr. Now to those who make $12/hr or are striving to get there please forgive me, but I'm having difficulty accepting that someone out there thinks my time is worth a measly $12/hr. I mean I made $70,000 last year, and now I'm going backwards. God, I don't mean to sound ungrateful. I mean some people have been looking for work for the last 6 months, and I haven't even been looking for 6 days and I have some promising interviews. I thank you for that. It's just...well let me shut up and stop complaining. He's opening a door for us to bring some money into this house so I am grateful for that. I didn't want to mention this because I didn't know if he'd be embarrassed about this. But for the past two weekends, hubby has been working a temp job that pays $11/hr. That's not the humiliating part. The bad part is that the job requires him to stand on the road, holding a sign. See there's a real estate and construction company that is building homes in a certain area and hubby has to hold a sign pointing people in the direction of these new homes. He said the job literally makes him feel like a bum on the street, but that's the only job he's been offered since he was let go in October. I know this has to be extremely difficult for him as well. I mean this is a man who made $150,000/year, and now he's holding a sign on the road for a few bucks. But right now we really can't be choosy. The mortgage needs to be paid. I'll let you know how the job thing goes. Hopefully I'll get offered another contract that is a little more appealing than what they're offering me now. Nevertheless, God's will be done; and I mean that with all my heart.

10:21 PM

I have to add this. Taylor was feeling kind of antsy so I decided to take her from hubby and put her on my lap while I was job hunting on the computer and she was playing with this little Mexican "noisemaker" I gave her. The thing has a handle almost like maracas, but the base above is shaped like a mini-drum. There are two strings on each side with beads attached so when you spin in back and forth it makes a cool little sound. Well I let Taylor play with this while sitting on my lap. All of a sudden she rears her little baby hand back and clobbers me square in the mouth. So now, I'm going to my interview with a fat lip.

W ell, needless to say, the interview went well and I was hired on the spot. It is official I am now an On-Site Supervisor/Account Executive for a staffing agency. Or in laymen's terms…I'm a Narc. It's my job to rat out the contractors on the client site that are not doing their work, or causing problems and such, so that they can be replaced, pronto.

It's Thanksgiving Eve and I had to work til 7:15 PM tonight. I can't complain because it's an easy job and I literally live 3 minutes away. I mean you can't beat that with a country stick. I can also, pretty much make my own hours as long as I don't work overtime. The turkey is in the oven, the potatoes are on the boil, and except for the fact that I'm sleepy, I feel pretty darn good. I may go into the office for a couple of hours tomorrow just to check to see how things are going. I may even take Taylor in there with me. Thank you God, for giving me an easy job, so close to my house. Lord, I thank you for allowing me to have a job at all in this economy. You are truly a lifesaver. When I think about it, it's pretty miraculous how things worked out. I didn't start actively looking for a job until Tuesday of last week and starting working on Monday of this week. That's pretty fast service, Lord. And if you recall, I prayed that God would grant me a job, but I also prayed that his will be done because I didn't know which job, was the best one for me, and I know he does. Well for such a time as this, the job I have is the job for me and I am grateful. And making $12//hr is a whole lot better than what I made before…two pieces of lint per hour.

Sunday, December 1, 2002 8:30 PM

*oday is the first day of the best days of my life. I keep telling myself this over and over, and even quoting it out loud, hoping one day, it's will sink in my brain, conscience and spirit to the point where I actually believe what I'm saying. It's not that I don't believe it on some level, but when things have been this bad, for this long, something has to break through to get things going in a positive direction again. I have to be honest though. I get a little weary of these positive affirmations, especially when weeks, months, and years start to pass. Because after a while you start to think, you're just saying this because you're supposed to. And you are because it really doesn't help the situation to speak the obvious in the case of a bad situation. As the proverb says, you are snared by the words of your mouth…and you are…I know this. Most people know this. But it's so much easier, and less risky to state the obvious. You get my point. Things are really bad. I don't see anyway out of this one. Life bites. All these statements just flow off the tongue for me right now because things aren't going as well as they could be. Money is tight. I'm so sick of saying that but I don't know what else to say right now. I guess I'll shut up now and pray that tomorrow will be a better day. I'm tired of saying that too. Peace.

I'm sure I must sound like a schizophrenic, but I'm going through major changes and adjustments during this phase of my life. Well, what I really want to say is that sometimes you really think you've got it bad, until you see someone in a worse situation than yourself. I am really grateful to have a healthy baby. I was talking to a guy today who has a son that has a severe heart condition. The little boy's heart is in such bad shape, the guy has to take him in for treatments at least once a week. When I talked to the guy today, I really felt stupid about the things I've been complaining about. Money isn't everything. I'm sure that little boy's family would trade any amount of money for their child not to suffer, and here I am with a beautiful, healthy daughter, complaining because I have bills and little money. I mean this guy has less money than I do, and I'm sure he has medical bills mounting up from the child's treatments…and his job may be ending any day now. I had to really ask God to forgive me for complaining, because things could always be much worse.

Tuesday, December 3, 2002 5:16 PM

❧

*I*t's been an interesting day, I guess you could say. It was a pretty slow day at work…which made it a little difficult for me because I was really, really sleepy. I came home for lunch to see Taylor. She really brightens my day no matter how things are going. Things were not bad actually today. We just don't have enough money for us to feed ourselves and Taylor. So Taylor's gets the most of whatever we have. I can go reapply for food stamps, but that's still going take about a week for them to even tell me if we qualify. But I'm not going to complain. We'll just eat what we have until I get paid in two days. Even then I still have to take all but $20 or so to pay on the mortgage, but that's how it goes. But I'm not going to complain.

Wednesday, December 4, 2002 6:59 PM

Today is another day.

Friday, December 6, 2002 7:11 PM

I guess I've lost my muse. I can't think of anything worth writing or talking about because I know you're tired of hearing me complain and so am I. I don't want to talk about work, or bills, or money or spouses, or children or nothing. I guess I my muse has left me. Hopefully it'll come back soon.

Saturday, December 7, 2002 4:02 AM

*M*y motto for the day is just do it! Don't talk about it don't think about it just go ahead and do it. And once you've made the decision to do it don't look back, just move forward. I've learned something about myself as I work this menial new job I have. I've learned that I don't want to be a psychologist, counselor, or a psychiatrist, because I don't like trying to solve people's problems. People make my head hurt!!! I don't mind listening but to try to solve people's problems is pretty stressful for me because I feel too much. What I mean is that it is so darn easy for me to take on other people's pain because I try to put myself in their shoes. I'm saying all that to say this. I've decided not to get a degree in psychology. I think I'm going to go ahead and get my MBA in marketing…especially as it relates to marketing psychology. I've always been interested in marketing and business; I just hate corporate America if that makes any sense. It's a red sky this evening and it looks beautiful. I remember my Dad saying, "Red sky in the morning sailor's warning, red sky at night sailor's delight." Which means tomorrow should be a beautiful day. By the way I wanted to talk a little about my Dad. He means a lot to me and I attribute ½ of all good things about me to him. One of the greatest things he taught me was perseverance. Not necessarily by his words, but always by his deeds. He has worked for the same entity for the past 32 almost, 33 years and it hasn't always been easy for him, but he stuck it out. He started out working outside as a land surveyor, and as he gained education, experience he worked his way up. Now he is the systems administrator for a very large portion of that entity. I don't ever recall him being late to work, nor do I remember him missing a day, unless he was on vacation. I'm very proud of who he is and what he has endured to make me who I am. My Dad is also a Vietnam Vet. Although he was the sole surviving son of my grandmother, he was drafted nonetheless. From my understanding, many of the young men who were drafted were sole-surviving sons, especially those of African descent. My Dad experienced many of the side effects of war, some physical and some emotional, but he didn't let that stop him from being the honest, responsible and honorable man he is. My Dad will be the first to tell you he has never been perfect, but given the tools he had, and the ones he didn't have, he was the best father he knew how to be. I give him much respect for that. I think the most amazing and life altering thing my father did for me was give me self –esteem. I will never forget as a teenager, going through the awkward stages of life, he once told me this. "You are an intelligent, attractive, and moral young woman, and any man in his right mind would give his right arm to be with you." Those words meant more to me than any thing at that particular time in my life and it set a solid foundation for my relationship with men. I became a woman who didn't have to have a man in my life to feel whole or complete, nor did I have to jump through hoops to keep one, because they just sort of came to me after that. Now some of them had to be sent on their way because they just weren't right for me; and some of them were just plain losers. But when the right one came along I knew it, and the funny thing about it my Dad knew it too, although he never told me until after we were married. I love my husband dearly, but because of my Dad, God forbid, we ever split up, as long as I have God, I'll be alright. It would hurt like heck, and my heart would be broken, but I would still be alright. Thanks, Daddy. And most of all thank God! But to anyone listening out there, if you have a daughter make sure you do everything in your power to ensure she has a relationship with her father, it will make all the difference in the world.

Wednesday, December 11, 2002 8:55 PM

✦

oday has been a hectic day. I had an interview with on of those staffing firms at 8:00 AM, I filled out an application, talked with the person from the office, and made a good impression I think…and still made it out of there and back to my office by 8:40 AM. I had to fire someone today it was not fun because the dude is a really cool guy. I just took him by his hand, led him away from every one else and broke the news to him. He took it well but there was still a bit of shock on his face. "I'm getting fired for speaking my mind?" He asked me. I took off my HR hat for a minute and said, "basically yes." It was not fun. I've never had to be the person to have to let someone go, and it's so close to Christmas. The decision-makers on the subject acted as if it was no big deal; they just asked me to make sure I led him off of the premises. This is the part of the job that is difficult. You have good people getting fired on the whims of one or two people, it just doesn't seem fair, and he's a brother on top of it. Lord knows in this job market, the powers that be would probably not choose a Black male for their key positions, especially when he/she runs into someone who reminds them of their daughter, sister, brother, or themselves. At least that's been my experience thus far. But I'm still young and my opinion may change. I was thinking of going home for Christmas, but that just ain't going to happen. Hubby's still interviewing as am I and we need every penny we can earn to go toward house-note, car-note, and the basic necessities of life. Peace, I'm outta here.

Thursday, December 12, 2002 12:49 PM

🦋

I'm actually here during the daytime hours. It's pretty…
uh…nice.

Saturday, December 14, 2002 12:59 PM

🦋

I just got in from work. Hubby says Taylor's been acting up. She probably just misses me. I mean, she's gone from seeing me everyday all day to only seeing me in the evening hours. I had to work today to make up some hours, because Lord knows I need the money. Taylor at least used to see me on Saturdays, but not today. Hubby was hired yesterday by a temp service that's offering an evening warehouse job. It pays $10/hr, a far cry from the six-figure salary he used to make, but we thank God for every single dollar. He's going to watch Taylor in the day while I'm at work and then he's going to work at night while I'm here with Taylor. I think it will work out well. It will take some adjusting on all of our parts. I think overall, it's a good plan to get some money in here to pay our bills, and not have to take Taylor to a daycare. Maybe when she turns two and we can afford a high quality daycare, we'll put her in then. Right now, I'm not feeling it. I have to call my brother today to tell him we're not going to make it home this Christmas, with so much going on money-wise, I think hubby and I should stay put. Well the muse has left me, as if it were ever there…

Wednesday, December 18, 2002 3:43 PM

This day will remain unrecorded.

Friday December 20, 2002 7:59 PM

This day will remain unrecorded.

Monday, December 23, 2002 7:43 PM

My baby is a year old today. It's so amazing. It seems like just yesterday she was born and I was in excruciating pain from the caesarean. But she's finally here, alive and well, healthy, brilliant, happy and full of life. She's the essence of my essence, embodied in a beautiful baby girl. I'm so grateful for Taylor… my miracle of miracles.

❦

*I*t's the night before Christmas and all through the house…naw, just kidding. Taylor is sleep for the night which is rare for her. Today was my last day as an onsite supervisor. I trained the new supervisor as best I could in the timeframe given. I think she'll be ok. I hope she'll be ok. A couple of the guys were giving her a hard time, talking about her English, because she's from Western Europe. She speaks perfect English as far as I'm concerned. They have to haze her like they did me, I guess. It's amazing how some of the people who I figured hated my guts were giving me hugs saying they hate to see me go…my how the tables turn. Hubby and I have done all the Christmas shopping we planned on doing. I basically just got things for Taylor. A few toys and some necessities like socks, shoes, and one cute little "snow princess" outfit. I'm actually going to miss all the people I worked with. It seems like I've worked with them a year, but it's only been a month. Time is funny that way. Well, I'm going to kick back and watch a movie…I might watch the Grinch first. Today has been a good day and I'm going to try to keep everyone of my former co-workers in my prayers.

🦋

I'm going through a lot of crap right now. I hope I don't offend the super-saint but I can only be myself at any given time and what you see is what you get. Thank God this year is about to end…I've had worse years so I'm not going to complain but this year in of itself has been a challenge. I've been having quite a scare for the past several days…I thought I was pregnant because I'm a few days late, and I'm never late. But I took a pregnancy test this morning and it was negative, which leads me to believe Hubby's theory, I'm just stressed to the nth degree and my body is responding accordingly. There are so many things up in the air in our lives right now and I wish we could just get them settled. We need stability…stability of income, stability in our quality of life, stability for our child. We literally do not get a break from the baby because we don't know people here in this state that we trust to watch the baby to give us a break. I would love to go to the movies with hubby; the last time we went together Taylor was about 3 months old and we became "that-couple-that-should-have-known-better-than-to-bring-an-infant-to-the-movies." But I feel their pain now that I'm a parent. You try to do things every so often to make yourself and your life feel normal again. Usually your attempts are futile, as was our trip to the theater. I was thinking today that I've been writing for 3 months now and I was hoping that something I said during the course of our stint together…would be of help to somebody out there. That's my whole purpose, to help someone endure the struggles of hard times whether they last 30 days or 30 years…I pray to God they don't last 30 years…but you know what I'm saying. Life can be really hard. It's hard when you have a spouse, it's hard when you don't have a spouse. It's hard when you have children, it's hard when you don't have children. It's hard when you have friends, it's hard when you don't have friends. The gist of the matter is this. Life can get so tough that unless a person is inside your brain at that particular time, it's difficult for them to understand the gravity of your plight. Well, I'm here to let you know that right here, right now, I am inside your brain and I completely understand. Hubby is at work tonight, I can't remember if I told you or not…he's working second shift in a Warehouse, making about 10 bucks an hour. He had me on the floor laughing when he told me what happened to him at work last week. Well, the first thing that happened was that he was talking to someone on the phone during his break and was taking notes on the conversation. He boss walked by and asked. "What you doing man, writing stories?" But wait, that ain't the funny part. He said the other day he was on break so he starting reading one of his books on Flash (it has something to do with building graphics on a website). He said this other dude walked by and asked, "What you doing man…you trying to learn or something?" It was hilarious. It was the equivalent of saying…"we don't allow no readin and writin around these parts." How sadly funny.

Tuesday, December 31, 2002 11:02 AM

It's New Year's Eve...thank God, I'm so looking forward to the end of this year and the start of 2003. 2002 has been a doosy. I'm grateful though; things are overall ok for the most part. We're all healthy, those been no major tragedies in my family and everybody's hanging in there. Nobody's lost their mind, gone on a shooting spree, robbed any banks, or sold their soul for a bowl of soup. We've made it...Thanks be to God...we made it! Hubby and I have been invited to a New Year's Party/Celebration, whatever you want to call it. Hubby can go but I'm used to bringing in the New Year with the Lord and not with a room full of intoxicated people. I'd like to go to communion tonight but I don't want to take Taylor out that time of night, so I'll wait til Sunday, when they usually have a "make-up communion" for those who didn't make it out New Year's Eve. 2003 is the Year of Unspeakable Joy! That's my declaration and affirmation for the Year. Talk at you later.

Today is the first day of 2003!!!!! Yippee! 2002 is over and done with. Praise the Lord. It was a hellish year. But this year is my year of Unspeakable joy; I'm going to affirm it everyday if I have to until circumstances catch up with my faith. Today I had quite an epiphany. I went to the track this morning for the first time in a long while. And my only intention was to run. I had a lot on my mind and I was just trying to clear my head and get my body and mind into the habit of running every morning. Well I started out on the track and I just took off running, and you know before I did, my mind does what it does every time I'm about to do something out of the ordinary, it starting making excuses for why I couldn't or shouldn't. "You remember you used to have asthma." "You're heavier than you ever been, you may break your leg running since you haven't ran with this much weight on you." Remember, you had a caesarean, what if your womb…" Then I did something I never ever do. I ignored all the little voices that told me why I shouldn't 'do something I really wanted to do and did it anyway. I just ran. I ran until I felt my legs burn. I ran until I felt like my ankles would break. I ran until my lungs felt like they would implode inside my chest. When I stopped I had ran ½ the length of the track. Then I walked again, fussing at myself for preventing myself from accomplishing all the goals I had set in life. Then I fussed at myself some more for not setting enough goals and settling for mediocrity in every aspect of my life. God did not allow me the privilege of living past all prognosis, to be just another grain of sand in the hourglass of time. I can and will make a significant mark on this world. I started walking to cool down and to keep my legs from collapsing (I'm exaggerating). Then when I got back to my starting marker on the track I took off running again. This time I started praying and asking God to give me balance in my life and help me do the things to maintain balance in my life. Then I asked him to help me use all the tools his given me to my advantage and simultaneously for his glory. I do want God to be pleased with my life. When I ran out of running gas again I stopped and looked up and I was at the same halfway mark as I was before. I did this one more time and with the same results. I ran out of gas at the halfway mark. At this point I began to get angry. How symbolic of my life my efforts to run today were. I keep doing the same thing expecting different results, which I'm told is the definition of insanity. On the 4th go-round I was down right mad. I wish I could have blamed the devil, but I couldn't. All this time in every stage of my life it has been one person preventing me from being great at something, anything. It was me. I'm the problem and today I was going to change that. I started running at the same point I had started 3 times before. But this time I did something different, I ran with sheer will-power and determination, because believe you me, at this point I was beyond exhausted. I also did something I very rarely do...I paced myself. Then it happened. God gave me a scripture from the Bible. "The race is not given to the swift, nor the battle to the strong, but to him that endureth to the end. I kept running, I was running at a 50-year-old joggers pace but I was still running. Then it hit me. I don't have to the prettiest, or the sexiest, or the smartest, or the fastest, or the slimmest, or the tallest, or the strongest. I just have to make it to the end. The end is every destination in every aspect of my life. I have now set goals for every aspect of my life and I'M GOING TO SEE THEM THROUGH. I got to the halfway mark this time and boy was I wore out, but I literally started calling on God to help me finish my little race. "The race is not given to the swift, nor the battle to the strong, but to him that endureth to the end." It was played over and over in my head like a tape recorder. I kept running. This was my life, and if I couldn't finish this little piddly made-up race I had set out to complete then what does that say of my life and my character, as a woman, as wife, as a mother, as a scholar, as a Believer. I would be pathetic. I kept running and I kept calling on God, until I literally felt a kamikaze sweep through my body and out of my feet. Then I was floating, I don't even know what caused me to look up, but I had not only passed the halfway mark, I had ran a full lap without stopping and working on my next lap. I laughed, I cried, I thanked God. Then I started walking, not because I was tired, not because I couldn't go any further, but simply because I had accomplished my goal and wanted to stroll on my victory lap and revel in the spoils of what God had done, and given me the strength to do. It was a beautiful day.

Thursday, January 2, 2003
🦋

*I*t's the second day of the year…so far so good. We found out today that Taylor is allergic to peanuts and /or honey. I made the mistake of listening to the pediatrician when they said that now that's Taylor is one, it's okay to give her eggs, peanut butter and honey. Bull-hockey. I gave her scrambled eggs yesterday and she did fine. But today I gave her graham crackers with a smidge of peanut butter and she broke out into hives. She starting scratching her face and rubbing her eyes…then I saw them. She had hives! Hubby got on the net to see what we should do about the hives. It said keep to keep her from getting hot and to put her in a tub of lukewarm water. I only saw hives on her face so I just kept putting a cold washcloth on her face. She thought it was a game and starting to perk up and laugh every time I put the cold cloth on her face. We did this about 50 times until I saw the hives go down. I then boiled her pacifier to remove any peanut butter residue. Then I put her on my lap with the pacifier in her mouth and begin to rock her to sleep, or so I thought. I heard this weird gurgle sound in Taylor's throat and then it happened. Everything she had eaten that morning came hurling up with a vengeance and the smell of old stomach juices. I mean I was covered from head to toe in spew and so was Taylor. I then, put her in the tub of luke-warm water like I should have done before and she splashed the water around as I washed her down. Then I removed her from the tub, dried her off and powdered her up, put her diaper on and at this point she had fallen asleep. I held her for a while as she slept, prayed over her once again and then put her down for her afternoon nap. It's a beautiful day.

*I*t's a beautiful day. I went running again this morning; I felt so refreshed afterwards. Once again there were only senior citizens on the track, but instead of the old man from the other day that I promise looked like Santa Claus in a leather jacket, there were some new people. There were two old ladies in orthopedic shoes and an old man walking in a jogging suit that had to have been a Christmas gift, because he looked so out of place wearing it. I have to renew my driver's license soon; I'm sure you could care less. I cleaned out my shelf today also that was stuffed with old papers and bills from yesteryear. I threw out everything that wasn't a necessity or had sentimental value. Taylor's crying because I put her in her playpen. I'm just afraid she's going to hurt herself because she's getting to the point where she's too fast for me. We don't have the stairs blocked off for monetary reasons and she hates when I shut the door to her room or my room so she can't wander to the hallway. I'm really using the wrong term. I'm looking for the word dart, so she can't dart into the hallway. Those little legs are faster than they look, so it's easy to misjudge how quickly she can get out of your reach. Well it appears that Taylor's crying has scared my muse away so I'll stop here.

Saturday, January 4, 2003 9:18 PM

This day will remain unrecorded.

Monday, January 6, 2003 9:06 AM

*Y*esterday was a good day. I went to church, got some strength, came home, ate and chilled out with Hubby while Taylor was sleep. We did nothing but talk, for about 5 hours straight, it was pretty cool. We didn't touch on the previous day's events...well at least I didn't, apparently it's hard for some people to let sleeping dogs lie. But you know what? I'm not going to sweat it. I learned at church today that you may not be able to change people, or the world around you, but you can change the way you look at things, which can only improve your quality of life. Hubby is quite a handful. As a matter of fact he's two handfuls, but I love him...what can I say? I love him. And no, I'm not trying to sound like some sort of wife martyr because I know I'm at <u>least</u> a couple of handfuls myself.

Tuesday, January 7, 2003 4:36 PM

❧

The house is pretty quiet…Taylor is asleep, Hubby is at work. It is very peaceful. I meant to mention this the other day, Hubby and I have decided that I would stay home with Taylor a little longer, since neither of us are comfortable with the whole babysitter or daycare thing…at least not until Taylor can communicate well enough for us to understand. That may not be for another year or so, but I feel good about it now that this part of our life is settled. Today is a decent day but I don't feel very inspired…so I'll catch you later.

*T*aylor has been fed, cleaned, and has had her hair brushed. All I need to do now is put her clothes on so maybe we'll go to the park . It's a beautiful day...I was supposed to get my hair done today, but when I got there for the appointment the salon was still closed. I guess they forgot that they made an 8:30 AM appointment with me...oh well...another day with my wig not up to par. I wanted to talk a little today about the state of the economy. Now I'm not siding with either of the major political parties because all have sinned and come short of the glory of God. But I think the President is definitely not the wisest man on earth, so if you didn't have your faith and confidence in God, you would probably be in a panic and for good reason. I mean let's talk about all the wars that our government has waged. War on Terrorism. War on Drugs. War on Iraq. War...War...War. I'm not a foreign or domestic political strategist, but the people here on the homefront are really suffering economically. Businesses are going under, families are losing their homes - things are really bad. But most people are oblivious to how bad things are because we don't talk to our neighbors like maybe our parents did back in the day. Things are worst than most people think, especially for middle class Americans. I'll get off my soapbox now. That little tidbit won't cost you a cent.

Thursday, January 9, 2003 11:51 AM

*F*inally!!!! I got my wig fixed this morning boy does my hair, head and scalp feel good. I have a phone interview today for a position that I'm actually interested in. I'll have the chance to run and operate my own office. I pretty psyched about it. I'll let you know how it goes.

Friday, January 10, 2003 1:46 PM

❧

*W*ell, the phone interview went well yesterday. Then the company had some location analyst (which sounds like a made up title to me) call me about a half-hour later. He was checking to see what my first and second choice for office locations were. So far, so good. They said the final step of interview process was to check my U-4 of course and then send me on to one last face-to face with one of the branch managers. I'm not as excited today as I was yesterday for the simple fact that we still don't have anyone we really, really trust to watch Taylor on a daily basis. Once again, I have mixed emotions about what once seemed to be a good opportunity. I talked to one of my old co-workers yesterday; she told me that things have pretty much went downhill since I left. Not to say that I was so irreplaceable or anything like that, things just got worse. I had a couple of weird dreams last night. One was that I got carjacked and the other was that two of my loved ones died. I chalk it up as me having a lot on my mind because I didn't eat anything before bed. This morning I took one of those IQ test, just for the fun of it. I guess deep down I like to be reminded that I am intelligent. I didn't do too shabby considering Taylor was running back and forth, whining and whatnot. I scored a 127, which is above average. My goal is to score close to a 200, which me rank me as the top 1% in intelligence. Based on the test I was categorized as an insightful linguist. They interpret that to mean that I have the natural fluency of a writer, and visual spatial strengths of and artist. I don't really know what to say about that, except this. How does that coincide with me being a financial advisor? It doesn't. You just have to do what you're trained to do to make money as you're working on your dream, which is what I am doing. It has been and always will be my dream to write something worth reading and hopefully I'm doing that now. I think I am, in fact. I went running this morning it felt good except now I'm a little sore. I gained about 6 lbs during the holidays and while I was working for 4 weeks. I've lost 2 of those lbs within the last week. I'm just having a meal replacement drink for breakfast, lunch and dinner and not eating after 7:00 PM. I'll let you know how it turns out. I'll tell you what I'll do from this point on. Every Thursday (except once a month when I'm bloated), I'll report my weight to you. This will hold me accountable and let you know my progress.

Saturday, January 11, 2003 11:05 AM

I'm pretty excited. Hubby and I are going to actually get to spend some time together without the baby. I can't even tell you how long it's been. I know its been several months. I don't know what we'll do, maybe go to the movies, go out for a cheap dinner. It doesn't really matter we just really, really need some alone time. A good friend of mine who is also a former co-worker said she would watch her for most of the day. She's watched Taylor several times before and so far has been the only no-relative to do so. I'm really excited, I have to find something nice to wear, and my hair is already done, so I don't have to do much to it. Yaaaaaaaaah!

Wednesday, January 15, 2003 12:20 PM

❦

*T*t's 12 noon and I feel good. I mean real good. This is the year of unspeakable joy and I feel it already. I bought Taylor some crayons today. I don't know yet if I regret doing so. She wrote on the couch and she looks like she's thinking about writing on the walls but hasn't done it yet, Thank God. Oh I meant to tell you Saturday was a heavenly day. I told you I had a good friend of mine watch Taylor and she did so for about 8 hours. Hubby and I went out for a movie, dinner, dessert at the bookstore and then dessert again. (smile). We had a ball. I don't know why I didn't have my friend watch Taylor before then…well I had her watch her twice before but there's something in me that hates to need anyone. Don't ask why, I really can't explain it all that well. All my life I have been one of those people who have always seen to the needs of others to the point that I ignored my own needs. I don't know if I have some inherent need to be the martyr, or that I'm just a power-freak, or that I just like helping people. Maybe it's a combination of all 3. I don't want to spew out too much psycho-babble. I just want you to know that I'm learning to let go of some of the things that have hurt me and one of those is letting the one person I trust to watch Taylor in this town, actually watch her from time to time. You know, so hubby and I can have some alone time.

Thursday, January 16, 2003 6:25 PM

O k. Yesterday I finished reading a really great book. It basically says that many of the problems we have in life coincide with our own bad attitudes, and what my uncle likes to call stinking thinking. One of the things that really hit home for me was the fact that many of us humans degrade ourselves on a regular basis. Now I have recently won the battle with speaking negatively about myself, but it didn't stop me from thinking negatively. How many times have we looked in the mirror and thought, "I look like crap." "I hate my hair." "My nose is too small/big/wide/flat/pig-like." Whatever the case may be. These are the thoughts that we think about ourselves so often, we don't even notice it. I've always complained about my hair, until yesterday. My hair was always something that I didn't want it to be - frizzy, dark, thin, kinky…the list goes on and on. But yesterday I started a new practice. I looked in the mirror and for the first time ever in my life, I said those seemingly forbidden words. "I love my hair." The first time I said it I looked around to see if anyone heard me, of course no one did because I was the only person within earshot. It's a good thing too because in our society, if you say anything positive about yourself you're considered conceited or arrogant. You're supposed to wait until someone else says something good about you, then and only then is it considered okay. After I said I love my hair about 15 times, I started something a little more daring. "I love my body." Man, oh man, I could hardly get the words out. I don't think I've ever said that in the history of my life…but I said that about 15 times as I looked in the mirror. It felt very uncomfortable at first then, something strange happened. It started to feel good. Then I did and said something that I promise you started a revolution in my own mind. I look in the mirror and said, "I love and accept you exactly the way you are." This was by far the most difficult for me, because like most people, I am my worst critic. But when I looked in the mirror and said those words over and over it truly did start a revolution in my mind. The tears began to well up in my eyes because I had never looked in the mirror and said anything close to that about myself. But let me tell you more about the revolution. I also started quoting other positive affirmations and backed them up with the Bible. "I am slender. I am completely healthy. I am prosperous." (I would that you prosper and be in good health even as your soul prospers…by his stripes we are healed.) "Wealth comes to me." (The wealth of the wicked is laid up for the righteous.) I just began to speak positively and think positively about everything that concerns me. That night I tossed and turned because my old mind, or old way of thinking begin to wrestle with my brand new mind/way of thinking. But thanks be to God, my new mind won out and I feel great. Oh by the way, it's Thursday and I weigh 187 pounds.

Friday, January 17, 2003 4:44 PM

O h, let me tell you all the crazy things that happened in the midst of my new positive thinking and speaking. 1. I went to pick up Taylor's pictures from the photographer and they had added some erroneous charges to my bill totaling $80 or so and it won't be cleared up for a few weeks according to the representative I spoke with. 2. I was told by a bill collector that we were being sued. 3. My final interview with the Financial Services firm is about 40 miles away, and I had to call her to set the appointment, and it's considered long-distance, and we didn't have long distance or a calling card at the time. 4. Hubby cashed his check from his temporary warehouse position and found out he was making $9.50/hr instead of the $10/hr he was promised. He had never checked his pay stub to see what they were paying him per hour. You see what I mean. As soon as I started speaking and thinking positively, things went haywire, in fact things started to get way worse than they were before. Now usually I would have gotten frustrated and cried and started speaking and thinking negatively again. But this time I didn't and it made all the difference in the world. Hubby got a new permanent position today. He starts Monday and we now have health and dental insurance and he makes $16/hr. Yippee! I am sooooooooooooooooooooooooo grateful to God for that.

✦

*I*n 10 days I'll be 33 years old. I thank God for every year I grow older, because many who have had my medical history have not made it this far. I was diagnosed with cancer for the first time 12 years ago. I had what the doctors called a "recurrence" 6 years ago. But for some reason God saw fit not to allow me to lose my breast, my mind, or my life. Thank you, God. Taylor is cutting more teeth so she is less than a happy camper. She wants me and her Dad to hold her, hold her, and hold her some more. I'm starting to miss my family, especially my brothers and sisters. I've also made the decision not to take the job with the financial services firm. I really don't want to be a Financial Advisor ever again, I was really thinking about doing it to help my brother. You see if I take the position, I will get to run my own branch office and I can hire whomever I like to be my assistant, on the company's dime of course. It's really a prestigious opportunity, outside-looking-in, but I'm really tired of doing things based on how it looks to others. I'm tired of impressing people. I've impressed people enough. Now I'm going to impress myself. As for my brother, I know he doesn't need me to give him a job to be okay. He's intelligent, resourceful, and talented. He'll be fine, I'll just continue to pray for him as I do all my family. We all need help right now. I really don't know if there's many of us who are really seeing their dreams come to fruition. I don't know if there are many of us who even have a dream. It's not a good feeling to not have a dream, I've been there. I had two dreams in my life. One was to be a model and the other was to be a published writer. In 1996 I was chosen as a finalist for an open call with a modeling agency, but I didn't follow through for many reasons. The first was that I was afraid. The second was that I had just gotten married and was worried how my marriage would be affected. Hubby encouraged me to go for it, nonetheless. The third was that I was still finishing up college and I felt that if I didn't finish then, I wouldn't finish at all. The fourth and final reason was that I spoke to someone who I really look up to and she advised me that Christians don't become models (I'm paraphrasing of course). All of these factors added up to me not pursuing the modeling dream and now that I have the gumption to do it, I'm 33 years old and a size 12. Not exactly what Cosmo is looking for, right. I am 5'8" though. That should count for something. Okay, now the being a published writer thing. I was always too afraid to go for it and I'll tell you one big reason why. MONEY. MONEY. MONEY. Most of the writers that I ever heard about were metaphorically and literally speaking…starving artist, at least starting out. Since I had made up my mind as a poor kid that I would not be a poor adult, being a writer was not in the cards for me. That's why I studied finance. My logic was that if I have a degree in money, I'd always have some, because I'd know what to do with it. Seemed like a simple plan at the time. So needless to say I didn't even try to write except when I was required to do so for some egomaniacal college professor. Another deterrent for me happened when

I was away at Governor Scholar Camp in high school. I volunteered to be on the newspaper staff and was asked to do a movie review. So I wrote what I thought was a masterpiece and submitted to the newspaper editor. When the paper came out I was so geeked about the whole idea, I grabbed a stack of copies. I looked for my review and it had been omitted entirely! Apparently someone did not agree with my review or either they questioned my writing ability altogether. I was so crushed I didn't even ask to see what the deal was. I just assumed I wasn't as good as I thought I was and stopped writing, or even talking about writing. I hope that little editor sees a copy of this book on the Best Sellers list. You know, not for revenge or anything like that…well, maybe a little bit.

Saturday, January 18, 2003 12:52 PM

🦋

I know it's still today, but I wanted to talk a little more. Not necessarily about anything in particular, I just have a lot to say today. I want to talk about my mother without going into too much detail because my mother is a very private person. You see I got it honest. I really love my mother, especially when I look at her through the eyes of the child I once was. She spent lots of quality time with me as she did all her children in their younger years. One of my fondest memories was when we used to take the bus downtown. I had to be about 3 or 4 because I wasn't in school yet...my older sister was. So while my Dad was at work and my sister was in school she and I would catch the city bus downtown (she didn't drive back then). We would do some window shopping on 4th Street and afterwards we would have lunch in one of those 5 and dime stores that also had a restaurant. I remember the first time she took me there for lunch, I ate the parsley on my plate, because I thought I was supposed to and I was always taught to clean my plate because of the children starving in Africa, or Bangledesh. So if they were starving, the least I could do is clean my plate, because somehow in my little mind, I felt that would help the situation. I chewed on the parsley while my mom was looking away and spit it out immediately. My mom turned around and laughed as she whispered, "That's for decora-

113

tion, you're not supposed to eat it." "Why would I need my food decorated?" I thought to myself. I also remember my mom giving me little crackers and Koolaid so I could have a tea-party with my teaset. But my favorite thing about Ma was that whenever I was sick, and back then it was quite often, she always let me lay in her bed. I mean, you could not lay in that bed for more than two days in a row without feeling better afterwards. I also remember whenever there was a bad storm, I would try to hold out, in my own room and bed until I heard the thunder. Once I heard the sky crack, it was curtains for any brave attempt to stay in my room. My sister and I shared a room but she always seemed to sleep right through the storm, which really ticked me off. How dare she get a good night sleep while I was sitting there petrified! Once I heard the thunder, my feet would grow wings and I would fly out of my bed, down the hallway, and take a dancer's leap only to land in the middle of both my parents. They never put me out…I was so grateful for that. My Mom has not had an easy life, but she always managed to keep a positive attitude, a trait that she passed on to me. I don't remember her ever being a complainer or a nag to us kids or my Dad (they're divorced now so he may beg to differ). She was as close as you could get to having Mary Poppins for a mother. As we kids started to grow up our relationship with my mother changed. For once in her life she started to do the things she wanted, whether they were good, bad, or ugly. We kids couldn't handle that. I mean we never looked at her as a human being who had hopes, dreams, and flaws. I mean, she was our Mother for crying out loud. Mother Nature, Mother Earth, Mother Teresa…Mother-May-I. She had been our mother since she was 15 years old and now she wanted to live her own life. How dare she. My mother had her mid-life crisis at 40, one husband, six children and one divorce later. I was 23 at the time but I took it really hard, you just never expect your parents to split up, I don't care who you are or how old you get. The 4 younger kids were split down the middle, the two boys with Dad, the two girls with Mom. Then they were split again, my baby brother with my Dad and my other brother and two sisters with my Mom. Then they were split again, my baby sister with my Mom, and my other sister with my Dad. The two boys were in college or on their own by this time. It's been 10 years and I still don't think my family has fully recovered. But I don't blame anyone because we all are victims or victors of the environment we were raised in. My parents both came from broken homes, so the fact that they made it through 25 years of marriage and 6 children is truly amazing. I've only been married 7 years and have 1 child, and I still have to call on Jesus from time to time. I am very proud of my mother, because she may not have had the best childhood, but she at least gave her heart and soul during mine. I know that may sound a little selfish…I don't mean it to be. But if she wasn't the mother to me that she had been, I would probably be dead. God always has a plan in the midst of chaos. She taught me to have faith in God. She taught me to think positively. She taught me not to wallow in depression. She taught me the scripture that saved my life. "He was wounded for my transgressions, he was bruised for my iniquities, the chastisement for my peace was upon him and with his stripes I am healed. I am healed. I am healed! I love you Ma…more than you'll ever know.

Sunday, January 19, 2003 6:10 P.M

🦋

*I*t's Sunday evening; the house is quiet. Taylor and hubby are taking a nap, so I can get away to write. I went church this morning, in spite of the fact that I lost one of my contacts when I fell asleep last night, and had to wear my glasses. Anyone that knows me, know that I never, but never wear my glasses in public, unless I'm doing something like running to the mailbox, or taking out the trash. I first got contacts during my senior year in high school, and except for a classmate who told me I looked like I hadn't slept for about 10 years, I got a very positive response. I guess every since then, since I had already spent 12 of my 18 years wearing glasses, I decided to only wear my glasses around the house. But this morning in spite of my hatred of glasses I wore them to church. If I hadn't, I wouldn't have been able to go because I can't see to drive, and in spite of hubby's good intentions the day before, he didn't want to go. So I left him here with Taylor while I ventured out with my "glassed identity." Taylor's awake now...we'll talk later.

Sunday, January 19, 2003 9:51 PM

🦋

*T*aylor kept whining today. It was really driving me nuts. I don't think I was cut out to hear whining of any sort for any length of time. I just can't handle it. I really have to call on Jesus because the crying truly rattles my cage. I just let hubby deal with her, this time. Now that I look back on things, that's probably why it took us so long to have child. Neither of us was really ready before now. I mean when I think about how demanding Taylor is with our time, I can't imagine trying to raise her with the lifestyle we had before. I mean we traveled all the time and both of us were really focused on having a career, or at least making a lot of money. Right now, the things we need I'm not sure money can fix. We need someone in our family to watch Taylor from time to time. The days, weeks and months on end with no breaks from her, really starts to take a toll. God help me.

Wednesday, January 22, 2003 9:49 AM

Tomorrow Taylor will be 13 months old. She's growing up right before my eyes. I don't have much else to say...bye for now.

Thursday, January 23, 2003 7:50 PM

It's Thursday and Taylor has really been active today. I mean really active. I really need to be a part of one of those "Mom's-Day-Out-Program's." But of course those cost money...it's only $100 a month or so but we don't have that to spare. I went ahead and sent off our paperwork to apply for foodstamps again. You remember last time they turned us down and right before Thanksgiving too. You remember...well even if you don't, I do. I talked a friend of mine today from back in the day. I was glad to know she and her family were doing ok. We became friends back when we were both about 10 years old. We had some crazy times. She lives in a totally different part of the country but she said they're feeling the effects of the economy as well as we are. This stupid war and Bushnomics are tearing the country apart in my opinion. You have the "Haves" against the "Have-Nots" against the "Used-to Haves." It's crazy, real crazy. Taylor is 13 months old today. Today was a very long day. Oh, we're also trying out one of those credit-counseling-agencies to help us get on top of things. It's funny. I used to advise people on what to do with their millions and now I'm trying to avoid bankruptcy, foreclosure, car-repo, liens and judgements. Funny was definitely the wrong choice of words. Ironic, it's all very ironic. Oh I'm supposed to report my weight today, you know, since it's Thursday. Today I weigh 188 pounds and that's including my "monthly bloat." Not too bad, huh? I think I'm going to start on my next book tomorrow. We'll call it <u>The Fat Journal.</u>

January 27, 2003 10:01 AM

🦋

I'm really in sort of a blah mood. It could be PMS, it could be the need for a nice long vacation, or a good babysitter, or both. I don't know, but all of that positive thinking and speaking has kinda gone out the window. I mean I haven't been speaking negatively, but I sure haven't been speaking positively. It's very difficult to do so when you feel like blah. Our dsl isn't working, so it's not like I can check e-mail or anything.

*T*oday is the day…the day I was born that is. I have lived on this earth 33 years and counting. Thank God we're still counting. I have to admit; I've been a little down in the dumps of late. Not because I'm turning another year older, because my philosophy on that is that as long as I look good and feel good, I really don't mind. Nor do I mind telling my age. I've been down because the financial situation is really wearing me down, we have bill collectors waiting to try to zap any source of income they can find, which is horrible. You just get to a point in your life when you get tired of struggling. I have struggled financially most of my life and it is no fun. I try my best not to complain because, and I know I sound like a broken record when I say this…things could always be worse. I really miss my family; I have to admit. Although, I don't want to move back to my hometown. I hated living there when I did, so that isn't an option. We need money and lots of it. And a steady stream of that will last long enough for our children's children to enjoy. Show me the money!!!!!!!!!!!!!!!!!

Thursday, January 30, 2003 8:55 PM

My birthday was pretty uneventful. All my peeps called me to wish me a happy one of course. I'm grateful to have loved-ones who care. Hubby bought me Chinese food and an ice cream cone. It was all he could afford, seeing he only had $10. I'm grateful for another year on this earth and no pain. My grandfather is dying of cancer right now. So is hubby's. Two butterflies about to be angels….I hate cancer.

❧

*M*y mother called to say that my Grandfather won't make it through the weekend. She and my uncle are headed to Ohio. I feel sad…I <u>did</u> get to spend time with him and I am grateful for that, in spite of the fact that I didn't meet him until around 20 years of age. I feel sad for Ma. That's her father and she just lost her mother 3 years ago. I can't even imagine. I expect that most people think their parents will always be around but as you enter your 30's you start to notice them aging right before your eyes. You see your parents start to take on the attributes of your grandparents, in spite of the fact that you're sure that they swore before cheese that they never would. It's inevitable. I love my Grandfather for the long weekend we spent together just two years ago. Who would have thought it be our last. I feel somewhat guilty because I hadn't called him that much during his bout with cancer. But what do you say to a dying man you hardly know. It just felt awkward. Forgive me Lord. I dedicate this passage to my Grandfather. I pray he goes painlessly and peacefully, as he prepares to meet his Maker. I love you Granddad.

Wednesday, February 18, 2003 12:16 PM

🦋

*H*ubby, Taylor and myself just returned from seeing my in-laws over the weekend. It was an interesting trip. By the way, my Grandfather passed away this past Saturday. I have to call my mom and check on her to see how she's holding up. He lived about a year and a half longer than they had first anticipated. Then when he became very ill this final time, he lived 6 days longer than they expected. My mother was able to say her good-byes, so I'm relieved of that. When we got to my in-laws, we found out that hubby's favorite great aunt had just passed away. We were both disappointed that she did not get to see Taylor in person. Hubby and I found out today that a business associate of his, that is as high as you can get on the food chain has upped and moved out of the country. We're both wondering if he knows something we don't as far as the "War with Iraq" is concerned. We are definitely living in interesting times and also very sad times. Death is all around us…but I'm reminded of the scripture that says, "a thousand shall fall at thy right hand and ten thousand at thy side, but it shall not come nigh thee." I'm standing on, by, in, and through the very word of God. Peace.

Monday, February 24, 2003 1:27 PM

*T*oday is a good day.

I know we haven't spoken in depth for a while, but I really haven't had much to say until today. I know I sound like a broken record, but I just want to know when things are going to turn around for us. Financially speaking that is. I received a job offer making somewhat decent money, but of course I had to turn it down due to the day-care for Taylor issue. It's not that I resent that fact, it's just that when you are barely making ends meet, you just want to do something, almost anything to change that situation. Then there's the issue of Taylor. (I'm just rambling as things come to me…there's really no rhyme or reason to the order that they're flowing.) Taylor is one of the most strong-willed, independent, bound-and-determined babies I have ever seen in my life. When she wants something she will do anything to get it, even if by doing so she hurts herself. That drives me crazy, because I want to be firm so that she doesn't think she can always have her way, but at the same time I want to protect her from hurting herself, and not restrain her in a way that she can't feel like a free individual. This parent-hood thing is not easy. There's only been one perfect child in the history of mankind and that was God's boy…Jesus Christ. I guess the people who said that parenthood was easy weren't doing it right or they weren't actually there to experience the "hood" part of it. It's sort of like knighthood.

You better have your armor on because you will face many battles and a few wars like the toddler years and the war of teenagery. I know that's not a real word, but you get my drift. I wish I had some assistance, because you need time away to regroup, replenish and re-strategize. Ma didn't tell me anything about this part. Calgon...take me away!!!!!!!!!

🦋

I have slacked off on writing because I really had not been truly inspired for quite a while. But today is different. I am inspired. I'm inspired to tell you about how sick I have been feeling of late, I mean I feel physically sick. Going to the doctor is not an option right now since we are without insurance. Taylor is covered but hubby and myself are not. Whenever I feel sick I take special care to pay special attention to my body. In some instances I've just had too much white sugar the day before, or too much salt, or it's a bug floating around. This time, I'm not really sure what it is but I don't like to be sick…I mean I don't think anyone does, but I really, really don't like to be sick. I've had enough sick days to last me a lifetime, thank you very much! I was pretty dizzy and nauseous this morning even though I had little or no white sugar or salt yesterday. When I was sick yesterday I figured maybe my blood pressure was up or something so I avoided salt all day. But this morning I woke up dizzy and nauseated once again. I don't think I'm pregnant and God knows I'm not ready for another baby any time soon, but given my health history, I'll take a baby over a long-term illness any day of the week. I was really sick to my stomach when I remembered something hubby's grandmother told me. She said eat something with a little salt in it to cure queasiness. So I ate a handful of chips after my cereal this morning and the queasiness went away. I really don't think I'm pregnant. My body just acts a little weird from time to time, like it's trying to get my attention, so I give it the attention it requires and I usually feel better after a few days. Taylor's being really good this morning, she's been playing and talking by herself; that makes me so proud. That's a sure sign that she progressing developmentally and just plain growing up.

March 5, 2003 9:27 AM

❦

Once again I have been banished to my own personal hell. This is the third time in my short life. I guess I should explain. Yesterday I found a lump or something in my breast. I noticed it a couple of weeks back but dismissed it attributing it to PMS. Well that cycle has ended and the nodule, lump, or whatever you want to call it is still there. It's about the size of a pea. Before when I have found lumps they are at least the size of a walnut or some other shelled nut. Over the past two months I've been telling people, Christians and non-Christians, of God's healing power and then I find a lump. This has happened to me before. I know it's the devil, trying to make a fool out of me. I actually don't feel foolish, I feel mad, real mad. I feel like what is wrong with my faith that each time I tell of God's healing power and that you can live a normal healthy life after breast cancer, here comes the ultimate curve ball. I must admit I didn't see this coming. Except for the fact that I have not been watching my diet like I know I should. I really have to ask God to give me more self-control because I'm so used to eating crap. Flavored potato chips, which are full of MSG. I also have consumed enough white sugar over the past six years to last a lifetime. I'm doing much better now, but fried foods were once a staple in my life. And I do have to take into consideration the time in my life when I was really depressed because I hated my career choice. That was a least two good years of chocolate overdosing. I really can't blame this one on the devil. I know what to eat and what not to eat to keep my body healed of cancer and I didn't practice enough self-control to adhere to what I know. But my prayer today God, is to help me to control my urge to eat junk. That means I cannot eat any more processed foods, red-meat, white sugar, white flour, foods laced with MSG, artificial-sweeteners, chocolate, and caffeine drinks. But I will eat lots and lots of fresh fruits, fresh vegetables, nuts, and fish on occasion. It's my own fault that this tumor is here. You know its funny. I clicked the T.V. on to one of the popular tele-evangelist one day. Now this is one that I rarely listen to. But this particular day at this particular moment he was talking about cancer. He said something very profound that I will never forget, and now that I think about it, it makes perfect sense. He said that you can have all the faith in the world to believe that God can and will heal your body of cancer. But if you continue to consume a pound of white sugar a day you will die of that cancer. He said you can have the faith to move mountains, and have a personal confession that God has healed your body, and through your awesome faith God will heal your body. But if you continue to eat fried-chicken and other fatty foods you will die of the cancer. You know I did not want to accept the words he gave, because if I did it would force me to begin to exert some personal self-control. As a Christian over time you learn to exercise certain self-controls. Let's take fornication and adultery for example. I know that if I don't put myself in compromising situations that I can avoid fornication or adultery. I know that if I don't surround myself with people who consume alcohol, I will never, even at my weakest point be tempted to consume alcohol. And the same goes for any vice that Christians strive to avoid; this I was taught from my youth up. But when it comes to food, we as Christians feel we can go hog-wild (no pun intended) because that is one of the few fleshly desires we can give in to that we think will not lead to sin. But to consume the foods in excess that you know are not good for your body is very similar to smoking a cigarette. You are slowly committing suicide. I can say this with honesty because in the depths of my depression I have eaten chocolate with the intent to hurt myself. I mean I would sit and eat a pound of chocolate in one sitting because the way I felt at that particular time, I wanted to die. It is very difficult to admit but it is true. For the past few years I have eaten in a way that I knew would lead to my death and I was okay with that because living seemed too hard. I would say from time to time. "I fought to stay alive for this." It wasn't that any person was treating me in a way that made me want to die, necessarily, it was the trials of life. That made me say, "forget this crap...pass the chocolate and the fried-chicken." I didn't realize this until just now as I began to write. Ladies and gentlemen, this is what you call an epiphany.

Saturday, March 8, 2003 12:20 PM

*T*his day will remain unrecorded...

Thursday, March 13, 2003 12:59 PM

This day will remain unrecorded..

Wednesday, March 19, 2003 10:06 AM

🦋

Today is the day. The day the U.S. is supposed to go to war with Iraq. Saying I am against the war is an understatement. I pray for the troops, seeing that many of them are teenagers and young people just beginning their lives. I pray for their spouses, parents and other relatives, who will be forced to worry about them for the next several weeks or months. I also pray for the President that God leads him, and that he actually listens. I know a handful of kids that are over there. Most of them were friends of my brothers and sisters. It's quite sad that they have to be willing to sacrifice their lives for what I believe is American greed. If Iraq was not as oil-rich as they are, would we be fighting this war? Probably not. I also think it's sickening that people who disagree with the war are being labeled anything from terrorist sympathizers to communist, to left-winged-nuts. I didn't vote for the President during the election because I didn't trust him. He reminded me of some of the stock-jockeys I used to work with. They'll say anything to get you to close the deal. And once you've committed they do whatever is in <u>their</u> best interest. I could be wrong about him; I've been wrong before…but usually my gut instinct is right on the money. Well enough about the President. I don't want to end up like the Dixie Chicks. The powers that be, sure know how to shut somebody up when they want to, don't they? I hate the fact that we're going to war. But I know God is ultimately in control of what goes on in this world and that if war ensues, he will work it out according to his sovereign plan. As Christians, we also have to take into consideration that certain events must transpire before the rapture. So be it, I just want to be sure I'm ready. I have a sense of foreboding about the whole situation. I don't think this war is going to be a walk in the park as many may think. 9/11 has proved that America is as vulnerable to an attack as any other country. The only difference is that this country has the means to defend itself.

Friday, March 21, 2003 11:42 AM

*T*oday is the first day of spring and the 3rd day of the war on Iraq. I hate war. The problem with war is that there is always someone who has to die. I have a problem with a person taking another person's life. That's just me. Last night we found out that hubby's so-called raise was not the whopping $9/hr increase that the company had promised…it's actually an increase of $1.97/hr. That makes a big difference. Needless to say I'm disappointed. I had already testified to one close friend about the increase and we were both thanking God together. I guess we're just thanking him in advance for the increase he will give. But I am grateful for the extra $1.97. Hubby was pretty upset about it; I on the other hand, was quite sad. I left last night to pick up some take-out for hubby and myself. Taylor had already eaten. Then all of a sudden I lost my appetite. While I was driving I started feeling some numbness, then an acute pain shooting up and down my left arm. There had been some pressure on the left side of my chest as well. All I remember thinking is, "I can't leave my baby here without me." She needs me. So I drove home and told hubby about the pain. He said it was stress and began to tell me things were going to get better. I sat there with no facial expression whatsoever as the pain, racked the left side of my body and the hot tears streamed down my face. "I've heard this before." I thought to myself. I'm not blaming him, because at this stage of the game he has little or no control over our destiny. The economy, the job-market, and the powers that be are dictating our lives. All of these factors, however, are subject to the "Highest Power." So we pray, work, and wait for things to change. It's the ultimate waiting game. I haven't been tracking my weight as I promised, nor have I been going running every morning like I was at the first of the year. However my weight to date is 185 lbs. I feel pretty confident about losing more, since I'm giving vegetarianism a try...for health reasons of course. I don't know exactly what's going on with my body, put I'm praying it's a false alarm like the many other times before. I'm also praying that this small lump, or whatever it is my left breast, just simply goes away. I have my semi-annual appointment with my oncologist at the end of next month. I also have my annual mammogram coming up in about four weeks. What a joy it is to have your breast fondled by a stranger, as it is maneuvered, only to be crushed between two very hard plastic plates. And then while the crushing ensues, you're told not to breathe or move. If we have the technology to build a missile that's designed to sniff out an enemy bomb, pin-point its exact locale and blow it smithereens, then why in-the-name-of-all-that-is-holy do I still have get my breast jammed between two plates to check for breast cancer?! It's ludicrous! Peace.

Tuesday, March 25, 2003 11:08 AM

🦋

I have scheduled my mammogram. The only catch is that I don't have any insurance. I'm too embarrassed to tell them that I don't have any insurance...

Thursday, March 27, 2003 1:19 PM

In case I forgot to tell you, hubby got fired from his job Monday. The details aren't really important. The end result is just that we are once again without income, blah, blah, blah. I'm really sick of talking about it so I won't. In light of the fact that there is a war going on in another part of the world and that many citizens, both foreign and domestic are losing their lives, or their loved ones; I will not complain. There has not been a day yet, that I have looked out my window to see bombs going off and I'm grateful for that. I don't have much else to say.

Tuesday, April 1, 2003 4:36 PM

❧

I was just sitting here playing solitaire on the computer, when I was suddenly inspired…okay, there goes my inspiration, Taylor is crying.

Wednesday, April 9, 2003 12:55 PM

O kay. I can't believe I'm about to say this, but we are seriously considering moving back to my hometown. I love to visit my hometown, because of family and friends. But there is a very good reason why I left. I HATED IT! I remember being so anxious to graduate from college so I could get out of town, for good. But now that the job-market has dried up here in the Dallas area, many people are grabbing their hats and headed for greener pastures.

Thursday, April 10, 2003 2:20 PM

I have to tell you...I've fallen off the healthy-eating wagon. Or shall I say I've been pushed off. It's pretty difficult to eat healthy when you have $40 to feed 3 people, as well as buy toiletries and diapers to last a week. So I'll hold off on my healthy diet until further notice. I'll keep you posted because I'm sure you're hanging on the edge of your seat. There are a lot of situations pending that I won't get into because I don't want to make my head hurt by thinking about them. So I won't.

Wednesday, June 11, 2003

🦋

*I*t's hump-day. I know it's been a while since we talked but I've been so busy and to be quite honest uninspired. I'm really trying to sort some things out. And what I'm finding is that there is no such thing as the perfect situation. There is no perfect job, there is no perfect spouse, there is no perfect house, there is no perfect child, there is no perfect city, there is no perfect country. I really just have to trust God that I'm in the best situation at any given time, because that is the situation that he has allowed me to be in. I have really been enlightened over the past few weeks…especially the past few days. I'm going to this training with my boss (of all people) and she has talked to us trainees about positive, personalized affirmations. This is just the healthy and logical response to all the negative thoughts and voices in your head. We all have them, whether it stems from our childhood or lifetime experiences. Whatever the cause, the voices are there. And no I'm not talking about the ones that tell mentally disturbed people to do mentally disturbed things, in fact I'm not even qualified to speak on that at this particular time because I don't have any experience in that area. But we all hear negative thoughts floating through our minds on the daily, much like the sound of our own voice. You know what? I am a writer. I feel so free and powerful and strong and intelligent and liberated and liberating when

I write. This is what I love to do. So how do I do what I love and still make money? I'm not sure yet, but I'm asking God constantly for the answer; I really need an answer. Hubby is still working on his music thing and things are looking much better than they have in a long time. And by the way I took a job about a month and a half ago, in the financial services industry and boy do I hate it. You know I really don't hate it, just like I don't really hate asparagus. But if you put asparagus in front of me and a pot of my mother's greens, I will choose the greens every time. Now I may add a few spears of asparagus on my plate just because I am a person that likes to mix things up. But my staple will always be greens when given a choice between the two. In this scenario, writing is greens, if you haven't figured it out already and asparagus is the financial services industry. My new job is very, very, very demanding, so what can I say except for the fact that I'm only writing because I am deliriously exhausted. Oh by the by…I went for my mammogram last week. They said everything was fine but I told them about the small lump I had been feeling in my breast. They didn't feel or see anything abnormal, but checked things out based on my history. They did a sonogram on my breast. It was kind of weird since last time I had a sonogram it was because we were checking to see Taylor (pre-partum). Well they moved the sonogram around my left breast and low and behold there it was on the screen in black and white. Thank God it only turned out to be a cyst (a sac filled with some disgusting yellow fluid that I insisted that they drain). They told me that there was no medical reason for them to drain it but when you've had breast cancer and the number of tumors I have had…you don't want to feel anything out of the ordinary when you do your breast exams. They say you should do them daily, but I do them weekly, just to make sure I'm not obsessing. Well I'm tired as heck. Be good.

Monday, July 07, 2003 4:53 PM

*T*oday is a great day!!! You know nothing has really changed as far as circumstances; we'll talk about that at another time. I just want to talk about the things that I am grateful to God for. I'm sooooo grateful to God that Taylor is completely healthy. She barely gets a sniffle. Then I think about myself. When I went in for my oncological check-up, one thing I noticed was that they had gutted out a whole section of the office, where a whole slew of examination rooms used to be. What they created in it's place, in my opinion, was quite creepy. It's a giant room that's completely open. And in it is a group of about 20-25 people all of which have IV's feeding them one of two things, either a chemo-cocktail or antibiotics to counteract the negative effects of the chemo-cocktail. What was even more disturbing was that most if not all of these people were at least 70 years old and very frail and feeble looking already. God only knows what they will look like or feel like, when the "treatment" is complete. So needless to say I am so grateful to God that my appointment was simply a routine check of my vitals and to confirm my cancer-free-ness. I have so much to thank God for, you just wouldn't believe it. Peace.

Monday, July 21, 2003 6:56 PM

Amen!

Friday, August 14, 2003 11:39 PM

✦

God told me to erase what I wrote on this day. So I did.

September 5, 2003, 7:23 PM

🦋

First…I'd like to give a shout out to my baby sis, who turned 22 today. I'm soooo proud of her. She's an independent young woman with a Bachelor's Degree in Accounting….Whoop! Whoop! Okay, I just wanted to say that I know it's been a long time since I wrote…I just have felt so very uninspired…and there have been a lot of things going wrong…1st we have 2 parties that are trying to foreclose on our home….don't ask me how we became so lucky to have 2…but somehow we've managed it! But I don't want to talk about that too much, which is also why I haven't wrote you in awhile. I'm just tired of rehashing the things that are horribly awry in my life…most of them, fortunately are just money problems. Money problems are by far, the easiest problems to overcome, because you can be sure that once you've taken a truckload of money and hoisted it toward the money problem-target (you know, with one of those giant medieval-sling-shot-cups), you can be certain that the problem will be blown to smithereens. So thank God I just have money problems! I don't have health problems…me and mine are in good health. I don't have drug problems…me and mine are drug-free. I could go on and on…there are so many things I can be grateful about, so many non-money problems that I don't have that could be plaguing each and every day of my life. Like for instance cancer…I know it's a recurring theme, but hey it's one of the few extremely bad non-money-problems that I have been acquainted with first hand. You notice I said acquainted with...cancer has been to me like that long lost distant relative that you meet for the first time, out of the blue, in the grocery store, or in my case on the college campus. And then once you've talked to the relative for about 30 seconds, you realize that you wish you'd never met them. But there's not a lot you can do, initially, because they are, in fact, a very ugly part of yourself.

Sunday, October 5, 2003 11:44 am

I was reflecting last night and the wee hours of this
morning on the words of wisdom I would leave behind
if this was my last day on earth….not that I think it is, because if it was I most definitely would not be sitting in front
of this computer, but that's a whole different story. I've lived
almost 34 years on this earth and if I had to name the top
ten lessons of life they would be this, well let's make it the
top eleven, because I've lived a full life:

1) Health is a gift from God….if you live a day without
   any physical pain….that is a blessed day.

2) You don't have to be born rich to die rich…and no I'm
   not talking about buying a million dollar insurance
   policy, if you can't afford one. I'm talking about how
   you can be a regular working Joe or Josephine and put
   the maximum contribution away in a 401k and IRA,
   invest the contributions properly and 25-35 years later,
   retire a millionaire.

3) Don't kill yourself going to a job. By all means go to
   your job, but come up with innovative ways to supple-
   ment your income, so that when the company folds, lays
   you off or hands you that cute little pink slip…(you've

already done number 2, so you do have emergency cash) you have developed whatever talent you have to make money and to take it to the next level, so that you can sustain yourself and your family, when times are tough, ie., the "Baby Bush Years."

4) Accommodate the shifts in life. There will be years of plenty and years of famine. Don't spend every penny you have in the years of plenty, so when the famine comes you have some things stashed away that you can fall back on. This deals with the financial, social, marital, and emotional shifts.

5) Parenting is hard. Anyone who tells you different, is a lie, and the truth ain't in 'em. Being a parent is the ultimate sacrifice of life. Sometimes we as women think having a child is having some novelty item that we can show off to family and friends. And we think it will fill some void in our lives that career and marriage did not. I have a news flash for you…your child will not fill that void! And you shouldn't expect him or her to….only you and God can fill the voids is your life, don't ever forget that. That's not to say that having a child is not fulfilling, it is very fulfilling, sometimes too fulfilling. That's why you'll see so many parents around mid August to early September, running around the department store, grabbing backpacks , blue jeans and notebooks while singing a rendition of "Happy Days are Here Again!" We all love our children more than we love ourselves, but understand that parenting is serious business.

6) Don't look your nose down on anyone…because you never know where life will take you. If you're rich or pseudo-rich, don't think your better than anyone…because in most instances your only one paycheck from poverty, one bad business deal from the pawn shop, and a few dozen stock-ticks from the soup kitchen. So treat everyone with decency and respect.

My problem was always looking down own people who used or abused drugs. I guess my judging them was based on the fact that I had had no experience with drugs, and the highlight of my experience with alcohol was when I was 10 and me and my older sister would take a couple of swigs of rum extract from the spice cabinet. But I digress, the crux of the matter is that I have learned that I have my own addictions, but, because they are not considered immoral, illegal, nor cause strange or erratic behavior, society deems them acceptable. Being the Southern woman that I am I am addicted to good food…I mean mac and cheese, home-made rolls, red velvet cake and ribeye steaks. I mean I'm addicted to the point that if you told me I had to eat rice and beans for the rest of my life and that I would still receive all the nutrients my body needed , I would go out kicking and screaming….that, my friends, is a problem….and since I know this is my problem I have to take it day by day one step at a time, and some days, ladies and gentlemen…I fall short. Spoken like a true addict….I'm working on it, and God has to help me to overcome.

7) I hate Corporate America…I mean to be quite honest, if I knew now what I was getting into when I was a poor college student working through the business curriculum, I would have simply walked away. But I had to do something that would make me feel like I wasn't wasting the good brains God gave me, and although basket-weaving and interpretive-finger-painting has always been more my style, I had to go get a Finance Degree. What a dummy! My advice is to study what you love and it will make you a healthier, happier, more balanced individual.

8) Everything, I mean everything, happens for a reason. When I think of the most horrendous experiences in my life, as I look back and them again and again…I see the hand of God guiding me down this intricate path called "my life."

9) "Ain't nothing that deep." I stole this phrase from Hubby…this is the phrase that will get you through if you ever get to the place you feel suicidal. Your whole world is crashing down around your ankles, your wife left you, the dog died, your friends turned their back on you, you got fired from your job, they're coming to get the house, car, and the furniture…and you feel like life just isn't worth living anymore, mainly because you're humiliated, alienated, isolated, and inundated. So you have thoughts of taking your life, but you think that will not go over well because you're a Christian. So what do you do instead…you pray for God to take you out of this world….because you're tired. My answer to you

is………."Ain't nothing that deep!" It's better for you to take an extended vacation that you really can't afford than to take your own life….ain't nothing that deep, ain't nothing that deep. AIN'T NOTHING THAT DEEP!!!!!

10) God is my source. He is the source of my financial security, He is the source of my analytical thinking, He is the source of me and my spouse's income; He is the source of my mental and emotional stability. He is the source of my happiness, joy and contentment... He is the source of my fertility, virility and vitality. He is the source of every good idea. He is the source of health and strength…ladies and gentlemen; the pressure is off…GOD IS MY SOURCE.

11) I am a survivor. I survived poverty, cancer, racism, sexism, ageism and other ism you can think of. I've survived broken hearts, shattered dreams and very, very severe reality checks. I've survived tumors and scar-tissue, surgeries and radiation. I've survived pollution and poison, asthma, steroids, head injuries and stitches. I've survived embarrassment, humiliation, persecution, bullies, witches, curses and ill-will. I have survived loss of sleep, loss of hair, loss of loved ones. I survived rude bosses, rude teachers, rude strangers and rude awakenings. I've survived prophesies and false-prophesies, jealousy and hatred from within and without. The most important thing I can tell you about me is that <u>I am a survivor</u>.

I was once a small, insignificant, wormlike creature, who was minding her own business, when all of a sudden I was summoned to a higher calling, embodied in sickness, pain, heartache and suffering. But now, I'm starting to feel the shell of my cocoon giving way. It's real tight in here, but I know any day now, whenever God says so, I going to bust out of this makeshift casket, because me and God are not ready for me to go home yet. And anyway, I want to try out these new wings…and see how far they take me.

About the Author

TONYA T. GRIFFIN was diagnosed with Stage II breast cancer at the age of 21, while pursuing her education at the University of Louisville in Kentucky. Although she followed most of her doctors' medical advice, she decided to forego chemotherapy to allow for a more holistic approach to fighting the disease. For the next 6 years she was cancer-free. But in 1997, at the age of 27, Tonya had a "recurrence." She again underwent a lumpectomy, and yet again refused chemotherapy.

Today, Tonya is a 36 year-old, 15-year, two-time breast cancer survivor. Since her first diagnosis, she has married her college sweetheart, received her Bachelor of Science in Business Finance, and given birth to 2 beautiful girls, ages 1 and 4 years old. Tonya's mantra for life is "He was wounded for my transgressions, He bruised for my iniquities, the chastisement of my peace was upon Him, and with His stripes I am healed."

Tonya uses various avenues to get the word out, that breast cancer is no longer just a middle-aged woman's disease. She also wants the medical community to begin to treat the "whole" person, when they are faced with a cancer diagnosis. Tonya says, "Cancer is a human disease, and she not just be treated in a test tube." Tonya works diligently as an advocate for survivors through various organizations, and her prayer is that all cancers will be eradicated in her lifetime.